Neue therapeutische Strategien in der hämatologischen Onkologie

Beiträge zur Onkologie
Contributions to Oncology

Band 36

Reihenherausgeber
S. Eckhardt, Budapest; *J. H. Holzner,* Wien;
G. A. Nagel, Göttingen

KARGER

Basel · München · Paris · London · New York · New Delhi · Bangkok · Singapore · Tokyo · Sydney

Symposium «Neue therapeutische Strategien in der hämatologischen Onkologie»,
Kiel, 3. September 1988

Neue therapeutische Strategien in der hämatologischen Onkologie

Bandherausgeber
H. Löffler; W. Gassmann, Kiel

26 Abbildungen und 23 Tabellen, 1989

KARGER

Basel · München · Paris · London · New York · New Delhi · Bangkok · Singapore · Tokyo · Sydney

Beiträge zur Onkologie
Contributions to Onkology

Dosierungsangaben von Medikamenten

Autoren und Herausgeber haben alle Anstrengungen unternommen, um sicherzustellen, daß Auswahl und Dosierungsangaben von Medikamenten im vorliegenden Text mit den aktuellen Vorschriften und der Praxis übereinstimmen. Trotzdem muß der Leser im Hinblick auf den Stand der Forschung, Änderungen staatlicher Gesetzgebungen und den ununterbrochenen Strom neuer Forschungsergebnisse bezüglich Medikamenteneinwirkung und Nebenwirkungen darauf aufmerksam gemacht werden, daß unbedingt bei jedem Medikament der Packungsprospekt konsultiert werden muß, um mögliche Änderungen im Hinblick auf die Indikation und Dosis nicht zu übersehen. Gleiches gilt für spezielle Warnungen und Vorsichtsmaßnahmen. Ganz besonders gilt dieser Hinweis für empfohlene neue und/oder nur selten gebrauchte Wirkstoffe.

Printed in Germany by Lipp GmbH, München
ISBN 3-8055-5046-4

Inhalt

Vorwort

In dem vorliegenden Buch sind die Vorträge des gemeinsamen Symposiums der Deutschen Gesellschaft für Hämatologie und Onkologie und der Arbeitsgemeinschaft Internistische Onkologie, «Neue therapeutische Strategien in der hämatologischen Onkologie», zusammengefaßt, das am 3.9.1988 in Kiel stattfand. Ziel der Tagung war es, den aktuellen Stand der Therapie der akuten Leukämien sowie der Non-Hodgkin-Lymphome zusammenzufassen und neuere Therapieverfahren wie ultrahochdosierte Chemotherapie, autologe und allogene Knochenmarktransplantationen sowie die therapeutischen Möglichkeiten zu diskutieren.

Unser Dank gilt den Referenten für ihre informativen Beiträge sowie Herrn Professor Dr. H. Bartels, Lübeck, Professor Dr. H.-P. Lohrmann, Lemgo, Professor Dr. J. Schubert, Bremerhaven, Professor Dr. W. Schneider, Düsseldorf, Professor Dr. H.-D. Bruhn, Kiel und Professor Dr. H. Illiger, Oldenburg, für die Moderation und Tagung.

Der Firma Heinrich Mack, Nachf., Illertissen, sei für die großzügige finanzielle Unterstützung, dem Karger-Verlag für die schnelle Drucklegung des Buches besonders gedankt.

H. Löffler
W. Gassmann

Beitr Onkol, vol. 36, pp. 1–10 (Karger, Basel 1989)

The Role of Maintenance Chemotherapy, Immunotherapy, Induction Dose Reduction in Elderly Patients and Double Induction in the Treatment of Adult Acute Myeloid Leukemia. Four Randomized Studies of the AML Cooperative Group[1]

Th. Büchner[a], W. Hiddemann[a], P. Koch[a], H. Pielken[a], D. Urbanitz[b], H. Kreutzmann[c], G. Maschmeyer[c], F. Wendt[c], R. Kuse[d], E. Thiel[e], W.D. Ludwig[e], H. Seibt[e], W. Gassmann[f], H. Löffler[f], C. Aul[g], A. Heyll[g], W. Schneider[g], R. Mertelsmann[h], C.H. Anders[i], M.R. Nowrousian[i], K. Straif[j], H.A. Vaupel[j], D. Hossfeld[k], K. Becker[k], A. Ho[l], H.H. Fülle[m], K.-P. Hellriegel[m], H.J. König[n], B. Emmerich[o], E. Lengfelder[p], W. Siegert[q], H. Bartels[r], J. Schwammborn[s], R. Donhuijsen-Ant[t], E. König[u], M. Planker[v], G. Middelhoff[v], K. Mainzer[w], K.-H. Zurborn[x], H. Köppler[y], L. Nowicki[z], W. Augener[aa], J. Karow[bb], M. Schroeder[cc], H. Eimermacher[dd], M.C. Sauerland[ee], A. Heinecke[cc] for the AML Cooperative Group

[a] Medizinische Universitätsklinik, Münster; [b] St. Bernward-Hospital, Hildesheim; [c] Evangelisches Krankenhaus, Essen-Werden; [d] Allgemeines Krankenhaus St. Georg; [e] Medizinische Universitätsklinik Steglitz; [f] Medizinische Universitätsklinik II, Kiel; [g] Medizinische Universitätsklinik, Düsseldorf; [h] Medizinische Universitätsklinik, Mainz; [i] Medizinische Universitätsklinik Tumorforschung, Essen; [j] Medizinische Universitätsklinik, Bonn; [k] Medizinische Universitätsklinik Hamburg; [l] Medizinische Universitätsklinik, Heidelberg; [m] Krankenhaus Moabit, Berlin; [n] Universitätsklinik, Erlangen; [o] Medizinische Klinik der TU, München; [p] Medizinische Universitätsklinik III, Mannheim; [q] Medizinische Universitätsklinik Charlottenburg, Berlin; [r] Medizinische Universitätsklinik, Lübeck; [s] Medizinische Universitätsklinik, Homburg; [t] St. Johannis-Hospital, Duisburg; [u] Medizinische Universitätsklinik Hämatologie, Essen; [v] Städtisches Krankenhaus, Krefeld; [w] Krankenhaus Altona, Hamburg; [x] Medizinische Universitätsklinik I, Kiel; [y] Medizinische Universitätsklinik, Marburg; [z] St. Franziskus-Hospital, Flensburg; [aa] St. Willehad Hospital, Wilhelmshaven; [bb] Städtische Krankenanstalten, Düren; [cc] Städtische Krankenanstalten, Duisburg; [dd] Städtische Kliniken, Hagen; [ee] Institut für Med. Informatik und Biomathematik, Münster

[1] Supported by grants No. 422-4001-01 ZP 01 23 and 8701 of the West German Bundesminister für Forschung und Technologie (BMFT).

Introduction

During the early 1970's, an important progress for the treatment of AML was achieved by inducing complete remissions in the majority of patients, thus opening the chance of long-term survival or even cure to at least a minority of patients. A further improvement of survival, however, did not clearly result from various post remission induction treatment concepts. In particular, the role of maintenance chemotherapy remained unclear as from the data of 8 representative multicenter trials published between 1981 and 1987 [5, 6, 9–12, 14, 15]. Furthermore, promising results from immunotherapy using high numbers of allogeneic, neuraminidase-treated blasts [1] had to be confirmed in a representative trial. For elderly patients a general induction dose reduction was recommended by others [8]. The optimum treatment in this age group, however, remained controversial. In younger patients more recently an improvement of remission duration has been attempted by various approaches of post remission induction intensification.

Objectives

Starting in 1978 the AML Cooperative Group has been conducting a series of multicenter studies in order

1. to objectivate the effect of the own TAD9 intensive induction regimen,
2. to establish the role of monthly myelosuppressive maintenance chemotherapy,
3. to analyze the effect of immunotherapy by intradermal injections of high numbers of allogeneic neuraminidase-treated leukemic blasts,
4. to analyze the effect of induction chemotherapy dose reduction in patients 60 years of age and older, and
5. to investigate the role of very early intensification by double induction in patients under the age of 60 years.

Study Design

Table 1 gives the design of the different randomized studies. The chemotherapy courses applied are given in table 2. In the 1981 study part B patients for immunotherapy received 10^{10} allogeneic neuraminidase-treated blasts by 48 intradermal injections monthly between the maintenance chemotherapy courses.

Table 1. Design of four multicenter studies of the AML Cooperative Group addressing the questions about the role of monthly myelosuppressive maintenance chemotherapy (1981 A), the role of monthly immunotherapy using allogeneic neuraminidase treated blasts (1981 B), the role of induction dose reduction in elderly patients (1985 60+ yrs) and the role of double induction in a recycling and in an alternating version (1985 16–59 yrs)

Study		Induction 1. Course	2. Course		Consolidation	Maintenance (3 Yrs)
1981 A		TAD9	(TAD9)*	R	TAD9	monthly one of AD/AT/AC
					TAD9	none
1981 B		TAD9	(TAD9)*	R	none	monthly one of AD/AT/AC
					none	monthly one of AD/AT/AC plus immunotherapy
1985 60+ yrs	R	TAD9	(TAD9)*		TAD9/DNR30	monthly one of AD/AT/AC
		TAD9/DNR30	(TAD9/DNR30)*			
1985 16–59 yrs	R	TAD9	TAD9**		TAD9	monthly one of AD/AT/AC
		TAD9	HAM**			

* second course if persistent blasts (conventional mostly one course induction)
** second course mandatory, starting day 21 (double induction)

Table 2. Chemotherapy courses applied in the 1981 and 1985 studies. TAD9/DNR 30 contains 30 mg/m^2 Daunorubicin on three days instead of 60 mg/m^2

TAD9	6-Thioguanine	100 mg/m^2 q 12 h orally	days 3–9
	Ara-C	100 mg/m^2/day continuous i.v. infusion	day 1 and 2
		100 mg/m^2 q 12 h 30 min i.v. infusion	days 3–8
	Daunorubicin	60 mg/m^2/day i.v. injection	days 3–5
HAM	Ara-C	3 g/m^2 q 12 h by 3 h i.v. infusion	days 1–3
	Mitoxantrone	10 mg/m^2/day 30 min i.v. infusion	days 3–5
AD	Ara-C	100 mg/m^2 q 12 h s.c. injection	days 1–5
	Daunorubicin	45 mg/m^2/day i.v. injection	days 3 and 4
AT	Ara-C	as in AD	
	6-Thioguanine	100 mg/m^2 q 12 h orally	days 1–5
AC	Ara-C	as in AD	
	Cyclophosphamid	1 g/m^2 i.v. injection	day 3

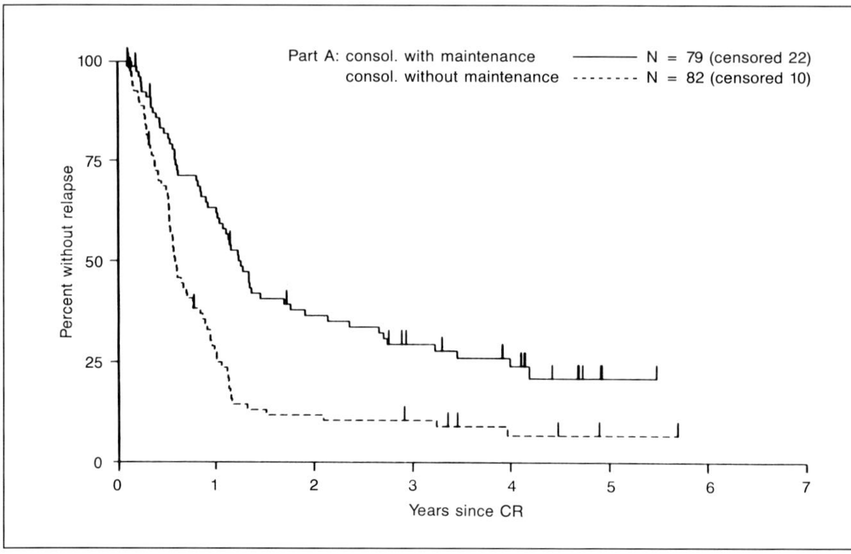

Fig. 1. 1981 study part A – Remission duration according to maintenance therapy ($p = 0.0001$). Tick marks represent patients censored in remission at last update. Patients censored in the first year include those receiving allogeneic bone marrow transplant (one in each group) or dying in remission during therapy induced aplasia (two in each group) or due to causes unrelated to treatment (two in the maintenance group).

Results

TAD9 Induction

Between 1978 and 1987, 1221 adult patients received TAD9 induction and were evaluable for response. A complete remission was achieved in 62.4% of the patients. In the 1978 and 1981 studies, 819 patients were treated according to the same induction strategy to possibly receiving one induction course only. CR was achieved in 61.5% with 68% of the remissions being induced by one course only.

Maintenance Chemotherapy

Remission duration in the 1981 study part A for patients randomized to receive or not receive monthly maintenance chemotherapy is given in figure 1. Figure 2 shows survival after relapse for the two groups. Treatment

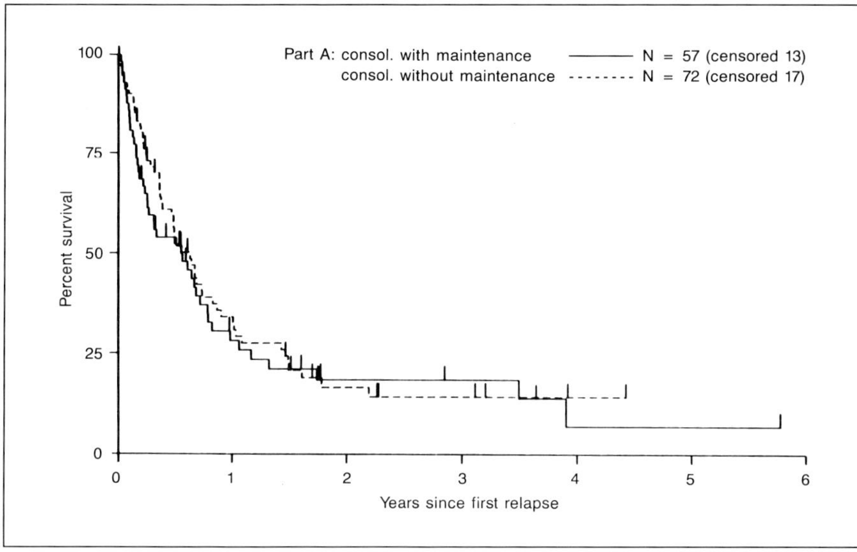

Fig. 2. 1981 study part A – survival after first relapse according to maintenance therapy. Tick marks represent patients alive at last update and patients censored at the time of bone marrow transplantation (6 in the maintenance and 5 in the non-maintenance group).

of relapse by protocol was a repetition of the primary induction regimen in patients relapsing after more than 6 months of first remission, and was optional in earlier relapses applying various second line regimens.

Immunotherapy

Remission duration in the 1981 study part B for patients randomized to receive monthly maintenance chemotherapy with or without immunotherapy is given by figure 3. No differences were found for survival after relapse for the two groups of patients. The same strategy was used for treatment of relapse as in part A.

Dose Reduction in Elderly Patients

For the 1985 study in patients 60 years of age and older response to induction is compared in table 3 between patients receiving TAD9 at full dose or at half dose for daunorubicin. For the two randomized groups total

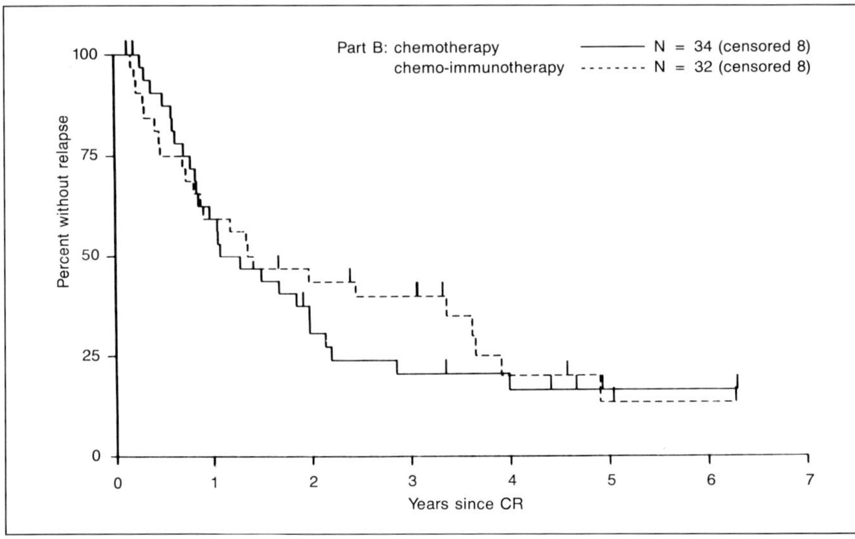

Fig. 3. 1981 study part B – Remission duration according to immunotherapy (p = 0.63). Tick marks represent patients censored in remission at last update and 2 patients dying early in remission (both in the group without immunotherapy).

Table 3. 1985 study in patients 60+ years of age. Response data according to TAD9 full dose vs reduced dose for daunorubicin

Induction	TAD9	TAD9 (DNR30)
Patients	42	51
CR	59.5%	43.1%
NR	21.4%	25.5%
ED	19.1%	31.4%

CR = complete remissions, NR = definite non responders,
ED = early death during first 6 weeks.

survival of all patients treated is compared in figure 4. There is no clear difference in remission duration between the two groups so far.

Double Induction

For the 1985 study in patients under the age of 60 years receiving two induction courses according to the double induction strategy the response

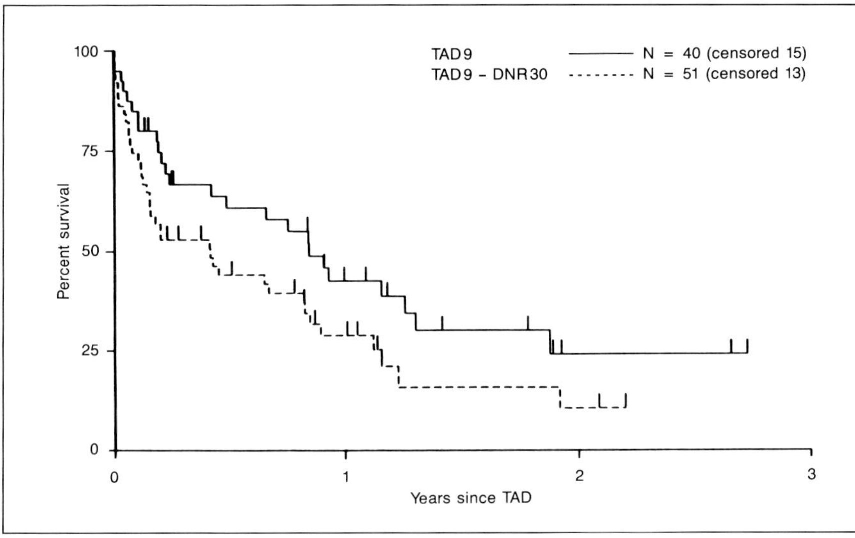

Fig. 4. 1985 study in patients 60+ years of age. Total survival according to daunorubicin dose reduction for all patients treated (p = 0.06). Tick marks represent patients alive at last update.

Table 4. Comparison of response to induction treatment in the 1981 (mostly single induction) study and the 1985 (double induction) study

Study	1981	1985
Patients	505	210
CR	64.1%	71.4%
NR	20.1%	16.2%
ED	15.81%	12.4%

CR = complete remissions, NR = definite non responders,
ED = early death during first 6 weeks.

data are given in table 4 and compared to the same age group in the 1981 study applying mostly one course induction. There are 76% CRs and 10% early deaths in the TAD9/HAM sequence versus 67% and 15% in the TAD9/TAD9 sequence. Figure 5 shows remission duration for the two randomized double induction sequences of the 1985 study.

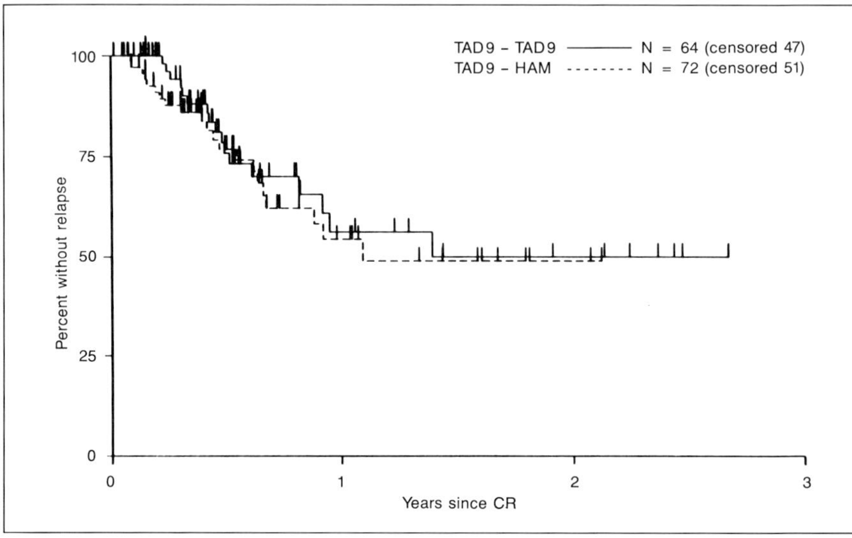

Fig. 5. 1985 study in patients 16–59 years of age. Remission duration according to the randomized sequence of double induction. Tick marks represent patients censored in remission at last update or patients censored at the time of bone marrow transplantation.

Discussion

The 1221 patients evaluable for response in our studies represent the largest number of adult patients with AML in multicenter trials. Furthermore, the 62.4% complete remissions in the entire group and the 61.5% CRs in the 918 patients treated according to an identical induction strategy have not been reached in another representative multicenter trial on adult patients of all ages not excluding very early deaths and defining CR by both bone marrow and peripheral blood criteria [5, 6, 9–12, 14, 15]. Thus, TAD9 represents a highly effective induction regimen for AML.

A clear evidence for the important role of post remission induction chemotherapy by consolidation and/or maintenance was obtained from our 1978 non-randomized pilot study [2, 3]. The important role of monthly myelosuppressive maintenance chemotherapy, still uncertain and controversial for many therapists, could clearly be substantiated by our 1981 study. Remission duration for the maintenance group in this study is among the best results of comparable trials together with one result from an almost identical maintenance regimen [10]. In addition, if analyzing remission duration in the 8 major multicenter trials and comparing patient groups with monthly or bimonthly myelosuppressive maintenance to those without comparable or any maintenance there is an obvious trend in favour of the maintenance groups. Those results lead our group to using maintenance as a basis for further improvement of AML treatment.

In contrast, immunotherapy using intradermal high numbers of allogeneic, neuraminidase-treated blasts failed to prolong remission duration. Thus, promising results from a mono-institutional trial [1] were not reproducable [13]. The uneffectiveness of this most consequent, experimentally based immunotherapeutic approach now allows to abandon immunotherapy of AML using leukemic cells and to concentrate on new immunological developments.

In elderly patients, the efficacy of induction treatment is limited by a higher early death rate in this age group. Some study results suggested that a dose reduction of induction regimens may improve response rates and reduce early death in elderly patients [8, 15]. However, in our 1985 study patients 60 years of age and older seem to benefit more from TAD9 at full dose than at reduced dose achieving a higher CR rate and a lower early death rate which also accounts for a longer overall survival.

The new strategy of double induction for the first time applies a second induction course routinely prior to achievement of CR. As from present early update this type of very early intensification may further improve remission duration. Double induction proved to be of good practicability when comparing the data of response and early death to those of the previous study applying a conventional induction strategy. This is especially true for the TAD9/HAM version introducing a high dose Ara-C/Mitoxantrone combination into primary induction treatment after having been sucessfully applied to refractory AML by our group [7].

On the basis of the effective strategies of double induction and monthly maintenance the treatment of AML may further be improved in the future by a more effective extended consolidation regimen.

References

1 Bekesi, J.G.; Holland, J.F.: Impact of specific immunotherapy in acute myelocytic leukemia, in Neth, Gallo, Hofschneider, Mannweiler, Modern Trends in Human Leukemia, Vol. 3, p. 79 (Springer, Berlin, New York 1979).

2 Büchner, Th.; Urbanitz, D., et al.: Longterm remission in acute myelogenous leukemia. Lancet *i:* 571 (1984).

3 Büchner, Th.; Urbanitz, D., et al.: Role of Chemotherapy for AML in remission. Lancet *i:* 1224 (1985).
4 Büchner, Th.; Urbanitz, D., et al.: Intensified induction and consolidation with or without maintenance chemotherapy for acute myeloid leukemia (AML): Two multicenter studies of the German AML Cooperative Group. J. clin. Oncol. *3:* 1583 (1985).
5 Cassileth, A.; Begg, C.B., et al.: A randomized study of the efficacy of consolidation therapy in adult acute non-lymphocytic leukemia. Blood *63:* 843 (1984).
6 Hayat, M.; Jehn, U., et al.: A randomized comparison of maintenance treatment with androgens, immunotherapy, and chemotherapy in adult acute myelogenous leukemia. A leukemia-lymphoma group trial of the EORTC. Cancer *58:* 617 (1986).
7 Hiddemann, W.; Kreutzmann, H., et al.: High-dose cytosine arabinoside and mitoxantrone: highly effective regimen in refractory acute myeloid leukemia. Blood *69:* 744 (1987).
8 Kahn, S.B.; Begg, C.B., et al.: Full dose versus attenuated dose daunorubicin, cytosine arabinoside, and 6-thioguanine in the treatment of acute non-lymphocytic leukemia in the elderly. J. clin. Oncol. *2:* 865 (1984).
9 Preisler, H.; Davis, R.B., et al.: Comparison of three remission induction regimens and two post induction strategies for the treatment of acute non-lymphocytic leukemia: a Cancer and Leukemia Group B study. Blood *69:* 1441 (1987).
10 Rai, K.R.; Holland, J.F., et al.: Treatment of acute myelocytic leukemia: A study by Cancer and Leukemia Group B. Blood *58:* 1203 (1981).
11 Rees, J.K.H.; Gray, R.G. et al.: Principal results of the Medical Research Council's 8th acute myeloid leukemia trial. Lancet *ii:* 1236 (1986).
12 Sauter, Ch.; Berchthold, W., et al.: Acute mylogenous leukemia: maintenance chemotherapy after early consolidation treatment does not prolong survival. Lancet *i:* 379 (1984).
13 Urbanitz, D.; Büchner, Th., et al.: Neuraminidase-treated allogeneic blasts for maintenance in acute myelogenous leukemia: results of a prospective randomized trial; in Büchner, Schellong, Hiddemann, Urbanitz, Ritter, Acute Leukemias, p. 64 (Springer, Berlin, New York 1987).
14 Vogler, W.R.; Winton, E.F., et al.: A randomized comparison of postremission therapy in acute myelogenous leukemia: a Southeastern Cancer Study Group trial. Blood *63:* 1039 (1984).
15 Yates, J.; Glidewell, O., et al.: Cytosine arabinoside with daunorubicin or adriamycin for therapy of acute myelocytic leukemia: a CALGB study. Blood *60:* 454 (1982).

Prof. Dr. Th. Büchner, Med. Klinik und Poliklinik, Innere Medizin A, Westf. Wilhelms-Universität, Albert-Schweitzer-Str. 33, D-4400 Münster (BRD)

Beitr Onkol, vol. 36, pp. 11–17 (Karger, Basel 1989)

Role of Consolidation Treatment with Increased Dosages of Cytosine Arabinoside in Patients with Acute Leukemia in First Remission

R. Willemze, W.G. Peters

Department of Hematology, Leiden University
Medical Center, Leiden, The Netherlands

Introduction

Cytosine arabinoside (Ara-C) is one of the most effective drugs for the treatment of acute myelogenous leukemia (AML). The success rate may be dose dependent since 10–30 mg/m^2 of the drug leads to remission in 10–50% of the previously untreated patients, whereas 100–200 mg is effective in approximately 30% of these cases. When the drug is administered in combination with an antracycline antibiotic with or without thiopurines complete remission can be achieved in 65–75% of the previously untreated patients [1–3]. The administration of higher dosages of Ara-C proved to be active in patients with relapsed and refractory leukemia [4–5]. The role of Ara-C in acute lymphoblastic leukemia (ALL) is less defined, although some studies suggest that increasing dosages of Ara-C might also be active in this type of leukemia [6]. The majority of the patients who achieved complete remission eventually relapses. Several investigators have administered high dose Ara-C as consolidation therapy to AML and ALL patients in first remission [7–12]. The results of these studies suggest that the duration of remission may be prolonged by such an approach. Autologous bone marrow transplantation is a new promising treatment modality available for consolidation treatment in patients with acute leukemia [13] and non Hodgkin's lymphoma in first remission [14]. Longterm disease free survival has been reported in 30–50% of the transplanted patients. A combination of those 2 intensive consolidation modalities is currently subject of several international studies. Between April 1982 and August 1988 we studied the effectiveness of high dose Ara-C and m-AMSA as consolidation therapy alone or in combination with autologues bone marrow transplantation for patients with poor risk AML and ALL in first remission. The results of this study are presented here.

Patients and Methods

Patients Characteristics

Between April 1982 and August 1988 we treated 44 adult patients with acute myelogenous leukemia and acute lymphoblastic leukemia in first remission. 24 patients were male and 22 female. The median age was 33 years (range 15 – 59). 17 patients reached a remission with standard induction therapy. 22 patients who failed to respond to standard remission induction therapy and 5 patients who developed AML after a preleukemic phase, received combination chemotherapy including Ara-C (1 g/m^2 q 12 h x 12) and m-AMSA (115 mg/m^2 for 1 – 3 days) and achieved a first remission.

Consolidation Schedule with High Dose Ara-C

All patients were eligible to receive 1 – 3 consolidation courses consisting of high dose Ara-C and m-AMSA. Cytosine arabinoside was given at the dose of 1 – 3 g/m^2, administered as 2 h infusion, twice daily for 4 days. In addition, m-AMSA (115 mg/m^2) was infused for 1 to 3 days.

Autologous Bone Marrow Transplantation

Bone marrow was harvested after the last consolidation course as soon as the peripheral blood values became normal, and the bone marrow showed a normal cellularity and a normal number of CFU-GM in the vitro bone marrow culture. After a conditioning regimen consisting of cyclophosphamide and total body irradiation (8 Gy) bone marrow cells containing more than 1 x 10^4 CFU-GM per kg bodyweight were infused.

Supportive Care

Supportive care was similar in all cases. Erythrocytes and random platelet transfusions were administered when indicated [15]. All patients were put on oral partial antibiotic digestive tract decontamination (1000 mg neomycin daily, 1000 mg amphotericine daily, 400 mg polymyxin daily and 2000 mg nalidixin acid daily [16]. They were cared for in single rooms, usually without flow facilities. Only those patients who underwent a bone marrow transplantation were nursed in rooms with down flow facilities. Mask and hand washing precautions were taken.

The duration of complete remission for patients was calculated from the recorded date of remission.

Table 1. High dose Ara-C consolidation in acute leukemia in first remission (Leyden Experience)

	No. of pats.	Sex f/m	Age mean (range)	Previously untreated	after preleukemia	Primarily failed	No. of consolidation courses	
							1 course	2 or 3 courses
AML	27	14/13	47(21–59)	11	5	11	16	11
ALL	17	6/11	25(15–48)	6	–	11	8	9
Total	44	20/24	30(15–59)	17	5	22	14	20

Results

The characteristics of the patients are given in table 1. Standard treatment for AML included standard dose Ara-C and daunorubicine, whereas standard treatment for ALL included vincristine, prednisone, daunorubicine and L-asparaginase. Patients who failed these treatment regimens and patients who developed an acute leukemia after a preleukemic phase received a course of high dose Ara-C and m-AMSA. Those who reached a complete remission are included in this study. 24 patients received only one consolidation course, 20 patients received 2 or 3 consolidation courses. The reason why patients received only 1 consolidation course was mainly because of undue toxicity. In 5 patients the reason was that the patients received an autologous bone marrow transplantation afterwards. Two patients died during the consolidation course, due to aspergillus septicemia and cerebral bleeding, respectively. The side effects of the high dose Ara-C consolidation courses are well known. They include drug fever (20%), fever due to local infection or septicemia (65%), skin rash (10%), ocular signs (15%), diarrhoea (10%), lung infiltrates (10%), and cerebellar toxicity (5%). The hematological toxicity consisting of a pancytopenia (granulocytes $<0.5 \times 10^9/l$, platelets $<10^9/l$) lasted a median of 19 days (range 16–21). The other side effects are described elsewhere in detail [17]. Exlcuding those patients who did not receive an autologous bone marrow transplantation, 9 out of 19 patients, who received only one consolidation course, relapsed, all of them in the bone marrow. Of those patients who received 2 or 3 consolidation courses only 5 out of 19 patients relapsed subsequently. One relapse presented in the skin, 1 in the central nervous system and concomitantly in the bone marrow. The other relapses were in the bone marrow. The interval from the date of remission to relapse in the group who received only one consolidation course was a mean of $6^1/_2$ months (range 3–11) and in the group of

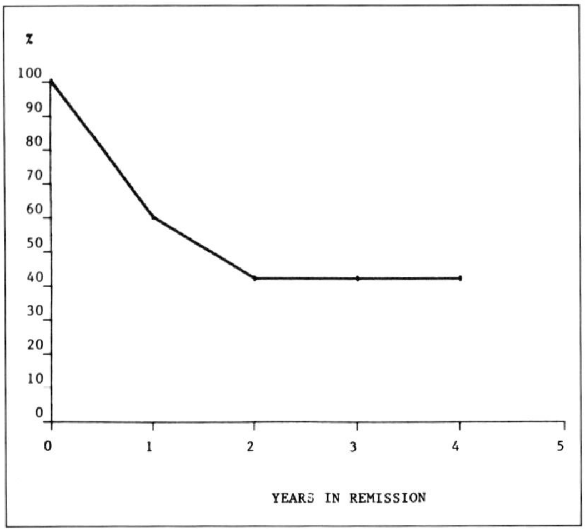

Fig. 1. Duration of complete remission in patients with acute leukemia in first remission, consolidated with a high dose Ara-C containing regimen.

patients who received 2 or 3 consolidation courses a mean of 17 months (range 5–24). The overall median duration of remission is 18 months (fig. 1) with 40% of the patients alive disease free after 3 years. Autologous bone marrow transplantation was performed in 6 patients with AML (3 male, 3 female). Bone marrow cells were immediately administered after the conditioning regimen, consisting of cyclophosphamide (60 mg/kg/dd, for 2 days) and total body irradiation (8 Gy). Granulocytes recovery was slow with a mean time of reaching more than 0.5, 1.0, 2.0 x 10^9/l granulocytes of 45, 65 and 117 days, respectively, and a mean time of thrombocytes to reach a situation in which platelets transfusion was not more required, or more than 50 x 10^9/l, and 100 x 10^9/l of 120, 179 and 215 days, respectively. At this moment, all transplanted patients are alive and well in a continuously complete remission for 3, 6, 12, 14, 40 and 41 months after achievement of complete remission.

Discussion

This report shows that long term remissions can be achieved in a considerable part of the patients with acute leukemia with intensive consolidation therapy including high dose Ara-C. The effect of high dose Ara-C as part of consolidation treatment in acute leukemia has been reported in the literature (table 2). High dose Ara-C consolidation therapy appears to result

Table 2. High dose Ara-C therapy after initial complete remission (CR) in acute leukemia

Other drug added	no. of patients	CR duration Median (Mo)	Long-term	Toxic deaths: No. (%)	References
Daunorubicin	25	30	38% at 2 yrs	1 (4%)	[7]
Daunorubicin	36	20	49% at 3 yrs	3 (8%)	[8]
Amsacrine	25	30	44% at 3 yrs	1 (4%)	[9]
Amsacrine	6	13	33% at 2 yrs	0 (0%)	[10]
	35	12	35% at 3 yrs	6 (17%)	[11]
Daunorubicin	33	23	50% at 3 yrs	4 (8%)	[12]
Amsacrine	38	18	40% at 3 yrs	2 (5%)	(this paper)
Total	204	21	41% at 2–3 yrs	17 (8%)	

in a substantially greater proportion of patients remaining in long-term remission than occurs after less intensive post-remission maintenance therapy programs where approximately 15% of patients remains in complete remission at 3 years. However, none of these trials was randomized, and in some there was substantial patient selection. For example, in one study median interval from remission to consolidation therapy was 3 months. Although these data with high dose Ara-C are encouraging, controlled trials are needed to confirm the positive impression.

More relapses occurred in our group of patients that received only one consolidation course. This finding is consistent with the results of Weinstein et al. [18], who showed that the addition of a number of intensive consolidation courses also increases remission duration. Since in spite of this intensive consolidation chemotherapy still many relapses occur, we started to study the possibility to combine the two most intensive consolidation regimens known in the treatment of acute leukemia, i.e. high dose Ara-C and autologous bone marrow transplantation. Our study shows that it is possible to harvest enough bone marrow cells immediately after several intensive chemotherapy courses and that the harvest bone marrow can be grafted after conditioning with a standard conditioning regimen (cyclophosphamide, TBI). However, hematological recovery, especially of the thrombocytes, is quite slow compared to the data reported in the literature [13]. This means that the requirement for thrombocytes transfusions is more intensive and lasts approximately 3–4 months. Whether the combination of high dose Ara-C and autologous bone marrow transplantation finally results in an increased chance of long term survival in these patients is not yet known since our study comprises of only 6 patients. This topic is subject of the new EORTC Leukemia Group Trial (LAM 8). The intensive consolidation chemotherapy has some serious side effects. Especially the high incidence of life threatening septicemia (mainly with streptococcus strains originating from the oral cavity or the digestive tract) was impressive. This could be explained by the more intensive mucosal damage after aggressive chemotherapy and the use of a decontamination protocol which selectively eliminated gram negative rods and staphylococcus aureus while leaving the anaerobic intestine flora and facultative streptococcus more or less untouched. The acute respiratory failure created serious problems. We suspect a relationship with Ara-C, as also has been suggested by others [19].

However, only 2 toxic death within 66 administered consolidation courses proves that the regimen is feasible, although in several patients a second course could not be given due to previously experienced life threatening toxicity.

Although based on non randomized trials, it is suggestive from our and several other studies that high dose Ara-C can be effective as consolidation chemotherapy for acute leukemia patients in first remission. The addition of autologous bone marrow transplantation after intensive chemotherapy is feasible although hematological recovery is delayed. Whether the combination of the two intensive consolidation modalities adds to the long term survival of the patient is unknown. A definite prove of its effectiveness must be provided by randomized trials.

References

1 Bodey, G.P.; Coltman, C.A.; Hewlett, J.S.; Freireich, E.J.: Progress in the treatment of adults with acute leukemia. Arch. Intern. Med. *136:* 1883–1388 (1976).

2 Cline, M.J.; Golde, D.W.; Billing, R.J., et al.: Acute leukemia: Biology and treatment. Ann. Intern. Med. *91:* 758–773 (1979).

3 Gale, R.P.: Advances in the treatment of acute myelogenous leukemia. New Engl. J. Med. *300:* 1189–1199 (1979).

4 Bollwell, B.J.; Cassileth, A.; Gale, R.P.: High dose cytarabine: a review. Leukemia *5:* 253–260 (1988).

5 Peters, W.G.; Willemze, R.; Colly, L.P.: Results of induction and consolidation treatment with intermediate and high-dose cytosine arabinoside and m-AMSA of patients with poor-risk acute myelogenous leukemia. Eur. J. Haematol. *40:* 198–204 (1988).

6 Peters, W.G.; Willemze, R.; Colly, L.P.: Intermediate and high-dose cytosine arabinoside-containing regimens for induction and consolidation therapy for patients with acute lymphoblastic leukemia and lymphoblastic non-Hodgkin's lymphoma. Semin. Oncol. *14:* 86–91 (1987).

7 Champlin, R.; Jacobs, R.; Gale, R.P.; Ho, W.; Selch, M.; Lanarsky, C.; Feig, S.A.: High dose cytarabine in consolidation chemotherapy or with bone marrow transplantation for patients with acute leukemia: preliminary results. Semin. Oncol. *12:* suppl. 3, pp. 190–195 (1985).

8 Wolff, S.N.; Marion, J.; Stein, R.S.; Flexner, J.M.; Lazarus, H.M.; Spitzer, T.R.; Philips, G.L.; Herzig, R.H.; Herzig, G.P.: High dose cytosine arabinoside and daunorubicin as consolidation therapy for acute lymphoblastic leukemia in first remission: a pilot study. Semin. Oncol. *12:* suppl. 3, pp. 1407–1411 (1985).

9 Vaughan, W.P.; Karp, J.E.; Burke, P.J.: Two-cycle timed sequential chemotherapy for adult acute nonlymphocytic leukemia. Blood *64:* 975–980 (1984).

10 Hines, H.D.; Mazza, J.J.; Oken, M.M.; Bennett, J.M.; Adelstein, D.J.; Keller, A.; O'Connell, M.J.: High dose cytosine arabinoside and m-AMSA induction and consolidation in patients with previously untreated de novo acute nonlymphocytic leukemia: phase I pilot study for the Eastern Cooperative Oncology Group. Semin. Oncol. *12:* suppl. 3, pp. 117–119 (1985).

11 Cassileth, P.A.; Begg, C.B.; Silber, R.; Spiers, A.; Burkhart, P.T.; Scharfman, W.; Knospe, W.; Bennett, J.M.; Mazza, J.J.; Oken, M.M.; Keller, A.M.; O'Connell, M.J.: Prolonged unmaintained remission after intensive consolidation therapy in adult acute nonlymphocytic leukemia. Cancer Treat. Rep. *71:* 137–14 (1987).

12 Tricot, G.; Boogaerts, M.A.; Vlietinck, R.; Emonds, M.P.; Verwilghen, R.L.: The role of intensive remission induction and consolidation therapy in patients with acute myeloid leukemia. Br. J. Haematol. *66:* 37–44 (1987).

13 Linch, D.C.; Burnett, A.K.: Clinical studies of ABMT in acute myeloid leukemia. Clin. Haematol. *15:* 167–186 (1986).

14 Verdonck, L.F.; Dekker, A.W.; van Kempen, M.L.: Intensive cytotoxic therapy followed by autologous bone marrow transplantation for non-Hodgkin's lymphoma of high-grade malignancy. Blood 65: 984–989 (1985).

15 Eernisse, J.G.; Brand, A.: Prevention of platelet refractoriness due to HLA antibodies by administration of leukocyte-poor blood components. Exp. Hematol. *9:* 77–83 (1981).

16 Guiot, H.F.L.; van der Meer, J.W.M.; van Furth, R.: Selective antimicrobial modulation of human microbial flora: infection prevention in patients with decreased host defense mechanisms by selective elimination of potentially pathogenic bacteria. J. Infect. Dis. *143:* 644–654 (1981).

17 Peters, W.G.; Willemze, R.; Colly, L.P.; Guiot, H.F.L.: Side effects of intermediate and high-dose cytosine arabinoside in the treatment of refractory or relapse acute leukaemia and non-Hodgkin's lymphoma. Neth. J. Med. *30:* 64–70 (1987).

18 Weinstein, H.J.; Mayer, R.J.; Rosenthal, D.S.: Chemotherapy for acute myelogenous leukaemia in children and adults. Blood *62:* 315–319 (1983).

19 Andersson, B.S.; Cogan, B.M.; Keating, M.J.; Estey, E.H.; McCredie, K.B.; Freireich, E.J.: Subacute pulmonary failure complicating therapy with high dose Ara-C in acute leukemia. Cancer *56:* 2181–2184 (1985).

R. Willemze, Department of Hematology, University Medical Center,
P.O. Box 9600, NL-2300 RC Leiden (The Netherlands)

Beitr Onkol, vol. 36, pp. 18–34 (Karger, Basel 1989)

Autologe Knochenmarktransplantation bei akuten Leukämien

Ergebnisse der Leipziger KMT-Gruppe – Internationaler Stand

Werner Helbig[a], Martin Kubel[a], Michael Wötzel[c], Franz-Albert Hoffmann[a], Helga Schwenke[a], Rainer Krahl[a], Volker Thierbach[c], Sabine Leiblein[a], Petra Feyer[b], Wolfram Pönisch[a], Elisabeth Schule[a], Brunhilde Haustein[a]

[a] Karl-Marx-Universität Leipzig, Klinik für Innere Medizin,
[b] Klinik für Radiologie und
[c] Bezirksinstitut für Blutspende- und Transfusionswesen Leipzig

Einleitung

Ermutigt durch die gegenüber der früheren konventionellen Chemotherapie akuter Leukämien (AL) günstigeren Langzeittherapie-Ergebnisse nach allogener Knochenmarktransplantation (KMT), wurde bei fehlenden histokompatiblen Geschwisterspendern vor etwa einem Jahrzehnt damit begonnen, die autologe Knochenmarktransplantation (AKMT) mit zumeist kryokonserviertem Mark aus der ersten oder zweiten kompletten Remission (CR) als Alternative im Rezidiv oder in CR 2, bald danach jedoch auch in CR 1 einzusetzen. Dies geschah, obwohl ein Rest leukämischer Stammzellen im Knochenmark anzunehmen und kein «graft versus leukemia»-Effekt (damals noch unsicher) zu erwarten war. Ermutigt durch günstige Ergebnisse von Pilotstudien an wahrscheinlich z. T. unbewußt selektionierten Patienten, aber auch durch eine relativ geringe «transplant-related mortality» (TRM), infolge fehlender «graft versus host»-Krankheit und der mit ihr häufig verbundenen Komplikationen, begannen besonders in Europa und den USA immer mehr KMT-Gruppen die AKMT einzuführen. Die höhere Rezidivrate führte trotzdem zu etwa gleichen Resultaten wie nach Allo-KMT; vielleicht auch deshalb, weil viele Gruppen früh begannen, den naheliegenden Gedanken einer In-vitro-Elimination von Restleukämiestammzellen, das Knochenmark-«purging», mit physikalischen (Zentrifugation), chemischen (Zytostatika) und immunologischen Methoden zu verwirklichen.

Ergebnisse der Leipziger KMT-Gruppe

Zwischen April 1981 und Juni 1988 wurde bei 48 Patienten mit AL (28 ALL in CR 1, 3 in >CR 1; 13 AML in CR 1, 4 in >CR 1) eine AKMT ohne «purging» vorgenommen (vgl. Tab. 1, 2). Alle Patienten erhielten nach CR 1 drei Konsolidierungszyklen mit Daunorubicin (45 mg/m^2 x 2), Cytosinarabinosid (100 mg/m^2, 2mal tägl. x 5 i.v.) und Prednisolon (60 mg/m^2 x 5), um eine weitere Leukämiezellreduktion zu erreichen. Die Erhaltungstherapie bestand rotierend aus monatlichen 5-Tage-Zyklen, die im 1. und 2. Monat ambulant (Vincristin, MTX, 6-MP bzw. Vincristin, Cyclophosphamid, 6-TG), im 3. Monat meist stationär (Daunorubicin, Cytosinarabinosid, bei ALL ergänzt durch Prednisolon) über 2 Jahre vorgenommen wurde.

Die Konditionierung erfolgte für ALL und AML durch Cyclophosphamid (60 mg/kg x 2) und Einzelganzkörperbestrahlung (TBI) mit 9,0–10 Gy; seit September 1987 für AML mit Busulfan (4 mg/kg x 4) und Cyclophosphamid (60 mg/kg x 4) nach Santos [27], für ALL durch fraktionierte TBI (2 x 2,0 Gy x 3) und Cyclophosphamid (60 mg/kg x 2).

An unmittelbaren AKMT-Komplikationen verstarben 5 von 48 Patienten (TRM = 10%) infolge Cardiotoxizität (3), Candidasepsis (1) und Hirnblutung (1).

Die hämatologische Rekonstitution war bei einigen Patienten verzögert, für Thrombozyten am stärksten. In Einzelfällen konnte keine völlige Thrombozyten-Normalisierung beobachtet werden.

Auch die Immunrekonstitution war nach einem Jahr noch nicht vollständig, obwohl die T-Lymphozyten bereits nach einem Monat den Normalbereich erreichten. Der T4/T8-Quotient fiel rasch ab und war häufig bis 3 Jahre nach AKMT erniedrigt; die LGL-Population jedoch erreichte schon nach 2–4 Wochen Normalwerte.

Die B-Lymphozyten begannen sich nach 2–3 Monaten zu normalisieren. Die Immunglobuline IgG und IgM blieben auch ohne Substitution noch im Normalbereich; IgA erreichte Basiswerte erst nach 2–4 Jahren.

Die Lymphozytentransformation durch Phythämagglutinin, Concanavallin A und Streptokokkenantigen normalisierte sich nach mehr als einem Jahr; gleiches gilt für die Hautteste mit Recallantigenen (Candida, Streptokokken, Tuberkulin).

Unter den Infektionen der immundefizienten Periode dominierten Virusinfekte, besonders durch Herpesviren. Außer Rezidiven wurden keine letalen Spätkomplikationen beobachtet. Die Wahrscheinlichkeit des «dis-

Tabelle 1. Ergebnisse der AKMT bei ALL

Literatur		n	Alter (range)	CR	Konditio-nierung	Pur-ging	Rezidive		DFS				MBZ (range)	TRM	
							n	(%)	n	(%)	%*	(Mon.)	(Mon.)	n	(%)
C.C. Anderson	[1]	8	27(16–49)	1	UCH	nein	5	(63)	1	(13)		–	32	3	(38)
S.J. Proctor	[25]	10	35(15–50)	1	Melph. + FTBI	nein	5	(50)		–	30	(36)	33(9–55)	0	
W. Helbig		28 3	23(15–39) 21(15–36)	1 >1	Cy + (F)TBI Cy + (F)TBI	nein nein	10 2	(36) (67)	14 1	(50) (33)	48 33	(72) (76)	29(5–72) 76	4 0	(14)
N. Ramsay	[26]	9 14	7(3–17) 9(6–17)	2 >2	Cy + FTBI Cy + FTBI	mo.AK mo.AK	15	(65)	7	(30)	29	(12)	21(6–32)	1	(4)
J.Y. Cahn	[4]	15	(12 Kinder)	1 + 2		Mafos. mo.AK	4	(27)	10	(67)	5>12 Mo.		– (2–45)	1	(7)
L. Mangoni	[20]	27	<50	1 + 2	Cy + (F)TBI	Mafos.		–			45	(54)			–
W. Santos	[28]	5 19	25(18–40) 18(3–40)	1 2	Cy + FTBI Cy + FTBI	4-HC 4-HC	2 16	(40) (84)	2 2	(40) (11)		– –	28(17–37) 41 (29–55)	1	(4)
M. Körbling	[18]	18	28(13–42)	1,2 + hr	FTBI + Cy	Mafos.	–			–	72		24	0	
P. Hervé	[12]	13	24(15–40)	1 (9) 2 (4)	TBI + Cy (30)	Mafos	4 (CR 1)	(44)	5 (CR 1)		(56)		28	–	
		23	8(3–14)	1 (2) 2 (21)	CT (6)	mo.AK	8/19	(42)	11/19		(58)		45	–	
B. Simonsson	[30]	54	–	1hr (21) 2,3 (32)	CT + (F)TBI	mo.AK	6 13	(29) (41)	– –		65 43		15 10	3	(6)

* berechnete Wahrscheinlichkeit, meist nach Kaplan-Meier.
CR: komplette Remission; CT: Chemotherapie ohne TBI; Abkzg. für Zytostatika; DFS: «disease-free survival»;
(F)TBI: fraktionierte und singuläre TBI; hr: «high risk»; Mafos.: Mafosfamide; MBZ: mittlere Beobachtungszeit; Melph.: Melphalan;
moAK: monoklonale Antikörper; TRM« «transplantation related mortality»; 4-HC: 4-Hydroperoxicyclophosphamide.

Tabelle 2. Ergebnisse der AKMT bei AML

Literatur		n	Alter (range)	CR	Konditionierung	Purging	Rezidive n	Rezidive (%)	DFS n	DFS (%)	DFS %*	DFS (Mon.)	MBZ (range) (Mon.)	TRM n	TRM (%)
P. Stewart	[31]	13	–	1	Cy + TBI	nein	8	(62)	3	(23)		–	(19–43)	–	
L.F. Verdonck	[34]	14	36(16–57)	1	Cy + TBI	nein	7	(50)	6	(43)	–	20	(6–43)	1	7
C.C. Anderson	[1]	16**	38(19–55)	1	CT (UCH)	nein	6	(38)	10	(63)	63	32	(24–69)	0	
A.K. Burnett	[3]	22	36(13–53)	1	CT + T(TBI)	nein	9	(41)	12	(55)	57(48)	27		–	
		90***	(10–57)	1	CT + TBI/CT	nein	27	(30)	–		56(36)			5	6
A.M. Carella	[5]	25	3815–51)	1	Cy + TBI	nein	6	(24)	13	(52)	~69	23	(8–49)	6	24
G. Meloni	[21]	15	10 (1–16)	1	CT (13 BAVC)	nein	7	(47)	8	(53)	–	>12	(n = 6)	0	
G. Meloni	[22]	18	27(0,9–52)	2	CT (BAVC)	nein	4	(22)	14	(78)	28	12	(1–40)	0	
W. Helbig		13	25(16–36)	1	Cy + TBI/Bu + Cy	nein	6	(47)	6	(46)	36	17	(2–64)	1	6
		4	24(19–28)	>1		nein	3	(75)	1	(25)	25	84		0	
J.Y. Cahn	[4]	18	24(3–44)	1	CT (TACC)	Mafos.	5	(28)	8	(44)	–	~22	(3–47)	5	28
W. Santos	[28]	5	17(15–32)	1	Bu + Cy	4-HC	1	(20)	3	(60)	–	7	(6–68)		
		32	27(4–54)	2	oder	4-HC	10	(31)	13	(41)	–	16	(1–41)	gering	
		10	31(19–54)	3	Cy + TBI (2)	4-HC	3	(30)	3	(30)	–	19	(18–60)		
L. Mangoni	[20]	21	<50	1 + 2	Bu + Cy	Mafos.CR	1<CR 2			–	52	~11	(–30)	–	
M. Körbling	[18]	17	22(17–50)	1	FTBI + Cy	Mafos.	–			–	68	12		7	19
		20		≧2	FTBI + Cy	Mafos.	–			–	50				
P. Hervé	[12]	28	– (3–45)	1	CT (TACC)/ FTBI + Cy	Mafos.	14	(50)	10	(36)	~60(TBI) ~25(CT)	– –		4	14

* berechnete Wahrscheinlichkeit, meist nach Kaplan-Meier.
** 8/8 mit Doppel-AKMT sind DFS
*** 14 Doppel-AKMT, multizentrische Untersuchung

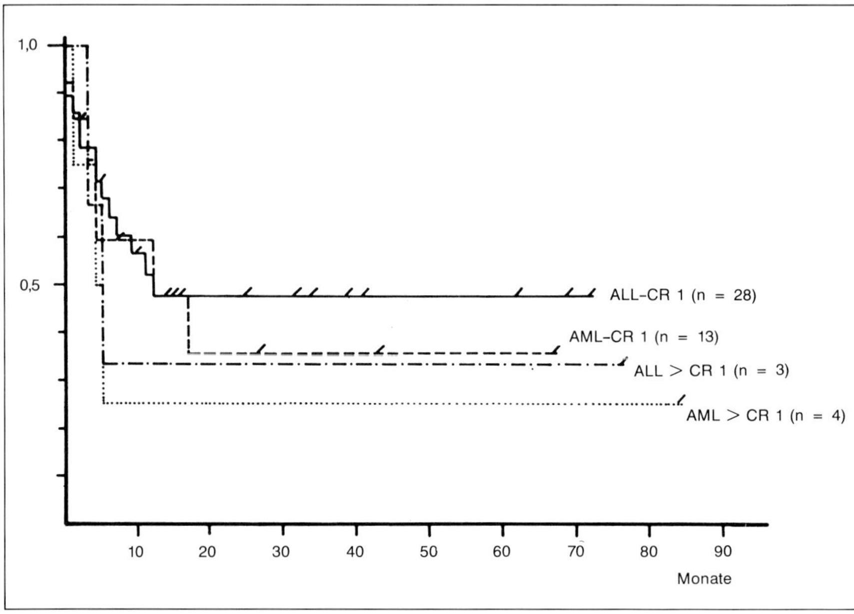

Abb. 1. Wahrscheinlichkeit des «disease-free-survival» (DFS) nach AKMT bei ALL und AML (KMT-Gruppe Leipzig).

ease free survival» (DFS) nach AKMT in CR 1 liegt für Patienten mit ALL bei 48%, mit AML bei nur 36% (Abb. 1), bei einer mittleren Beboachtungszeit (MBZ) von 29 bzw. 17 Monaten. Die 10 Rezidive bei ALL ereigneten sich im Mittel nach 6 (1–12) Monaten; 8 Rezidive bei AML nach 4 (1–17) Monaten.

Von den 7 jenseits der CR 1 transplantierten AL-Patienten rezidivierten 5, alle zwischen 1 und 5 Monaten.

Patienten mit einer Induktionstherapiedauer von mehr als 3 Monaten bis zur CR 1, als einem Indikator der Leukämiezellsensitivität, wiesen nach AKMT im Gegensatz zu solchen mit einer Therapiedauer bis zu 3 Monaten ein schlechteres DFS ($p<0{,}01$, Abb. 2) und «overall survival» (OS; $p<0{,}005$) sowie mehr Rezidive ($p<0{,}025$) auf.

Von den 21 nach AKMT rezidivierten Patienten (2 regenerierten mit leukämischer Hämatopoese) verstarben 7 innerhalb von 2 Monaten, im Mittel nach 4 (1–20) Monaten. 5 Patienten erreichten eine neuerliche CR (alle in CR 1 transplantiert); eine Patientin mit ALL lebt 54 Monate nach AKMT in CR 3. Somit unterscheiden sich die Wahrscheinlichkeiten für DFS und

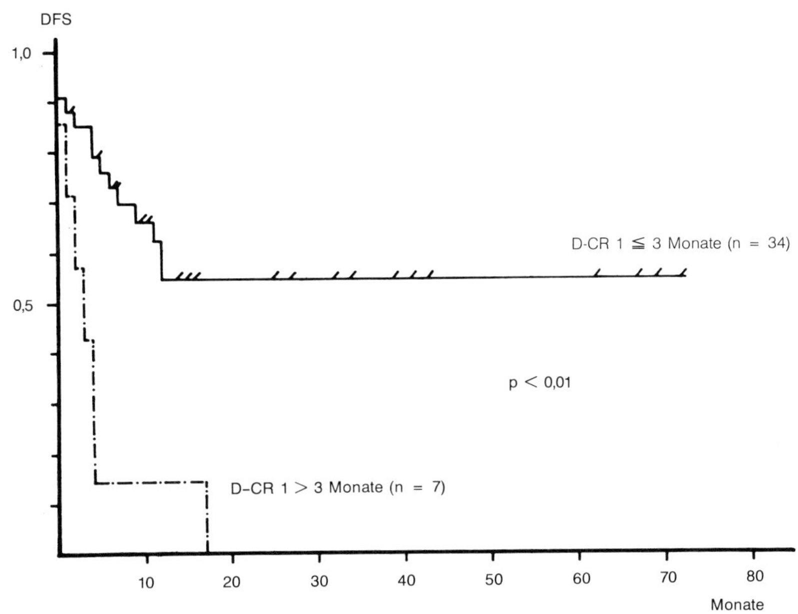

Abb. 2. Wahrscheinlichkeit des DFS nach AKMT für Patienten mit ALL und AML, die die CR 1 nach 3 bzw. mehr Monaten Induktionstherapie erreichten (KMT-Gruppe Leipzig).

OS (Abb. 3) praktisch nicht. Auf weitere analytische Resultate wird im letzten Abschnitt Bezug genommen.

Internationaler Stand

Unter Berücksichtigung von internationalen und eigenen Ergebnissen läßt sich für die AKMT bei ALL (Tab. 1) bzw. AML (Tab. 2) feststellen:

1. Die TRM liegt mit im Mittel 6 (0–38)% meist niedriger als bei KMT, wahrscheinlich aber höher als bei konventioneller Chemotherapie nach CR 1.

2. Rezidive sind unter Berücksichtigung der z. T. kurzen MBZ häufiger als bei KMT, auch mit gepurgtem Mark.

3. Das DFS ist, abgesehen von allgemeinen klinischen Parametern wie bei der KMT, abhängig vom Erkrankungsstadium, wahrscheinlich auch von der Art der Initialbehandlung inkl. der Postremissionstherapie, von der Leu-

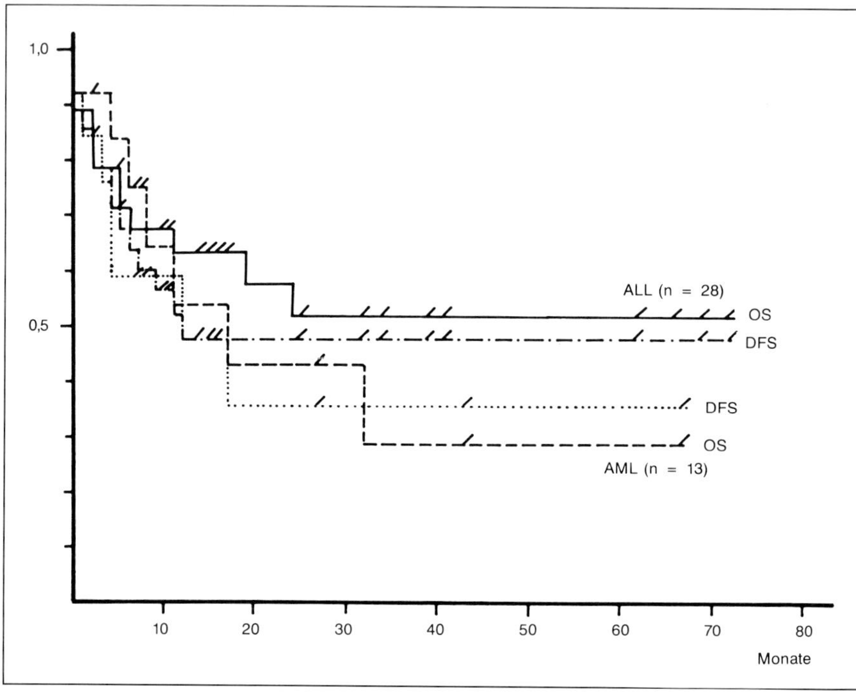

Abb. 3. Wahrscheinlichkeit des «disease-free-survival» (DFS) und des «overall survival» (OS) nach AKMT bei ALL und AML (KMT-Gruppe Leipzig).

kämiestammzellintensivität, von der Konditionierung und vom «purging»-Verfahren.

4. Die allgemeine Beurteilbarkeit ist infolge kleiner Patientenzahlen mit z.T. kurzer MBZ begrenzt.

Durch internationale Registraturen, besonders die Europäische KMT-Gruppe (EBMTG), können infolge multizentrischer Analysen genauere Aussagen erfolgen [9–11]. In nur drei Jahren stieg die Beteiligung von 30 auf 50 Zentren und von 380 auf 976 bewertbare AL-Fälle an (Tab. 3). Während das DFS bei AKMT in CR 1 und unverändertem In-vitro-«purging»-Anteil des Autotransplantates in dieser Zeit für ALL-Patienten von 48% auf 40% kaum zurückgeht, vermindert sich, bei nur zu etwa ein Drittel gepurgten Autotransplantaten bei AML-Patienten das DFS von 48% über 40% auf 34% (für die Gesamtpopulation) nach 75 Monaten. Für die in CR 2 Autotransplantierten besteht nunmehr bei ALL Erwachsene zu 20%, bei Kin-

Tabelle 3. AKMT bei AL (EBMTG-Analysen nach [9–11])

	1986	1987	1988
Zentren (n)	30	38	50
ALL/AML (n)	168/212	285/338	436/540
ALL/AML-Purg. (%)	71/38	72/34	71/?
ALL (DFS %/Mo.)			
CR 1-std.	48/36	42/56	40/60
CR 2	nicht diff.	35/56*	33/20–45**
AML DFS %/Mo.)			
CR 1-std.	48/48	42/70	34/75***
CR 2	35/12	40/40	32/40

DFS: «disease-free survival»; std: Standardrisiko
* Kinder 38%/56 Mo.; Erwachsene 10%; p = 0,05
** Kinder 40%/45 Mo.; Erwachsene 20%/20 Mo.
*** Gesamtpopulation; nicht nur std-Patienten

Tabelle 4. AKMT bei AL: «purging». EBMTG-Analysen nach [9–11])

1986	1987	1988
ALL-CR 1: Mafos./∅: 68/43% DFP (ns)	ALL-CR 1: Mafos./∅: 58/30% DFS (p = 0,1)	ALL-CR 1 – poor risk: Mafos/mo.AK: 63/39% DFS (p = 0,06) Mafos. ind./mo.AK: 82/40% DFS (p<0,05)
AML: keine Diff.	AML: keine Diff.	AML-CR 1 – std.: Mafos./∅: 52/30% DFS (p = 0,1) Mafos. ind./∅: 64/35% DFS (p<0,01) nach TBI: Mafos./∅: 56/32% DFS (p = 0,02)

DFP(S): «disease free probability (survival)»; Mafos.: Mafosamide;
mo.AK: monoklonale Antikörper;
TBI: Ganzkörperbestrahlung; ind.: individuell eingestellt

dern zu 40% die Wahrscheinlichkeit eines rezidivfreien Überlebens; für AML-CR 2 wurden 32% ermittelt.

Die letzte EBMTG-Analyse zum «purging» vor AKMT [11] erbrachte für den Mafosfamide-Einsatz erstmals einen Vorteil bei AML-CR 1, jedoch nur für die Standardrisikogruppe und besonders bei Strahlenkonditionierung bzw. individueller Mafosfamidedosierung (Tab. 4). Für Patienten mit ALL in CR 1 konnte nur in der poor-risk Gruppe eine Überlegenheit des Purgings mit Mafosfamide gegenüber monoklonalen Antikörpern (mo AK) ermittelt werden. Weitere Belege oder Trends [11] wurden trotz offenbar vielfältiger Computeranalysen nicht beschrieben.

Offene Fragen

Die häufig aufgeworfene Frage nach dem Einfluß der Dauer zwischen CR 1 und Knochenmarkentnahme bzw. AKMT auf das Ergebnis wurde ebenfalls kürzlich von der EBMTG durch Gorin et al. [11] untersucht. Patienten mit AML-CR 1 und AKMT nach ≦3 bzw. 4–9 und >9 Monaten nach CR 1 hatten ein DFS von 26% gegenüber 40% und 65%. Für ALL-CR 1-Patienten lagen die Relationen ähnlich (Abb. 4). Im Gegensatz dazu liegt das DFS für die ≦3 Monate nach CR 1 in Leipzig autotransplantierten Patienten günstiger als für die nach 4–6 Monaten transplantierten, obgleich die Unterschiede bei kleiner Fallzahl nicht signifikant sind (Abb. 5) und sich die Rezidivwahrscheinlichkeit genau umgekehrt verhielt. In Übereinstimmung mit der Schlußfolgerung von Gorin et al. [11] bekräftigt dieser Befund unsere Arbeitshypothese eines zumindest partiellen In-vitro-«purging» durch Konsolidierung. Umgekehrt ist die Frage zu wiederholen, ob Patienten, die erst nach 7 Monaten zur AKMT kommen, noch des «purging» bedürfen [11] bzw. überhaupt noch autotransplantiert werden sollten.

Bei den «purging»-Methoden sind die in vitro wirksamen Cyclophosphamidderivate wie Mafosfamide bzw. 4 HC [4, 8, 12, 18, 20, 28, 35] und moAK gegen Lymphozytensubpopulationen [4, 7, 12, 26, 30] klinisch am häufigsten eingesetzt worden und deshalb schon recht gut zu beurteilen (vgl. Tab. 1, 2). Für das Immuno-«purging» sind durch bessere moAK und Methoden [6, 16], so durch die «Immunobead»-Technik auf Magnet- oder «floating»-Basis [6, 13, 23], für das Chemo-«purging» durch die Kombination von Zytostatika, z.B. Mafosfamide mit VP 16 [5] bzw. die kombinierte Anwendung mit moAK [15] günstigere Resultate zu erwarten. An weiteren «purging»-Möglichkeiten z.B. mit Alkyllysophospholipiden [24], Merocya-

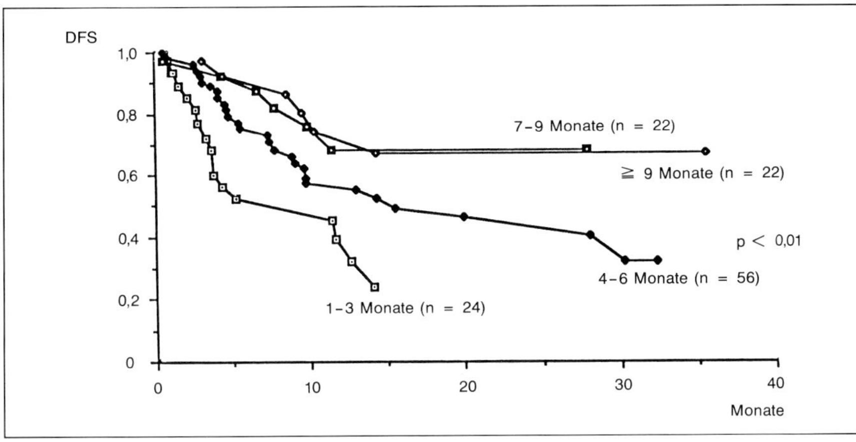

Abb. 4. Wahrscheinlichkeit des DFS nach AKMT bei ALL in differenten Zeitintervallen nach CR 1 bei ALL (EBMTG; Gorin et al.; Mitteilung an Studienteilnehmer).

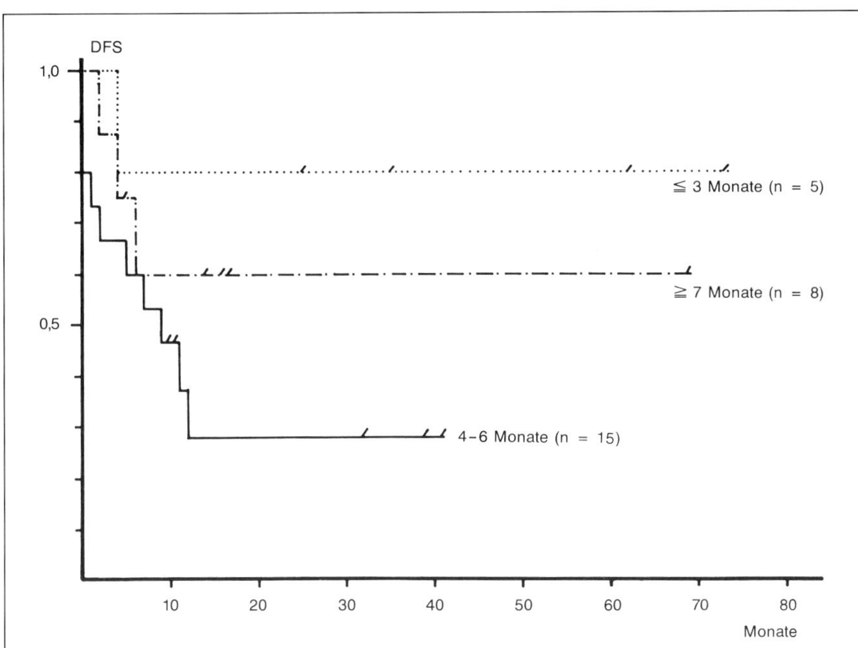

Abb. 5. Wahrscheinlichkeit des DFS nach AKMT bei ALL in differenten Zeitintervallen nach CR 1 (KMT-Gruppe Leipzig).

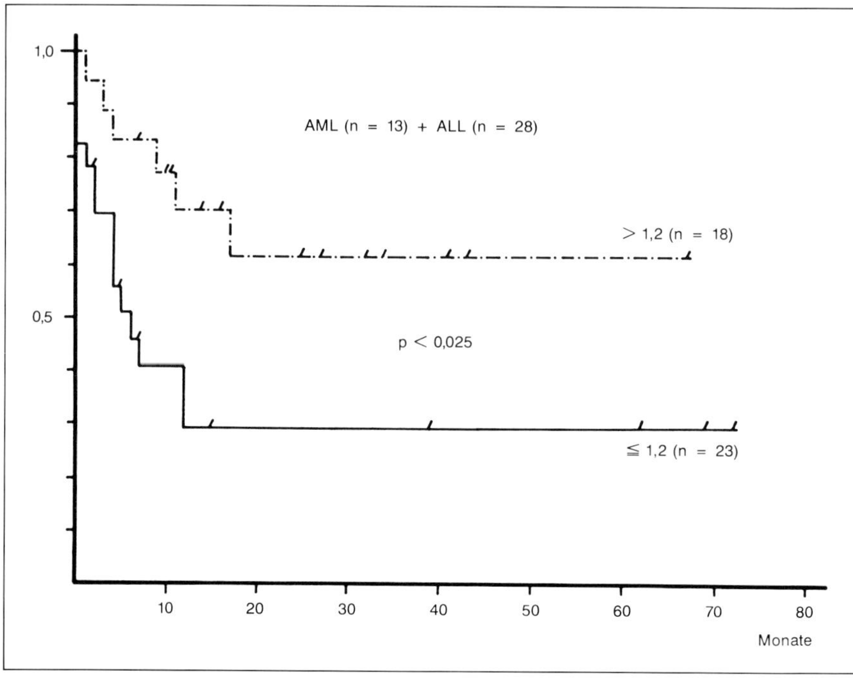

Abb. 6. DFS-Wahrscheinlichkeit in Abhängigkeit vom Gesamt-Mitose-Index des Autotransplantates bei ALL plus AML (KMT-Gruppe Leipzig).

Tabelle 5. Möglichkeiten zur Erkennung maligner Resttumorzellen (nach [15])

Konventionelle Morphologie	2–5 %
Einzel-Marker-Analyse (evtl. mit FACS)	0,5–2 %
Ig- oder T-Cell Rezeptor Gen. Rearrangement	1–2 %
Doppel-Marker mit TRITC/FITC-Labelling	0,2–1 %
Doppel-Marker mit nukleärer TdT	0,02–0,1 %
Klonierungsteste für ausgewählte Lymphome	0,001 %

nin-vermittelter Photolyse [29] und sogar Lymphokin-aktivierten Killer (LAK)-Zellen [19, 32] wird gearbeitet.

Ob die autologe Blutstammzelltransplantation eine echte Alternative zur AKMT bei AL werden kann [17, 33], vielleicht sogar infolge eines geringeren Leukämiezellgehaltes mit weniger Rezidiven einhergeht, ist derzeit ebenfalls offen.

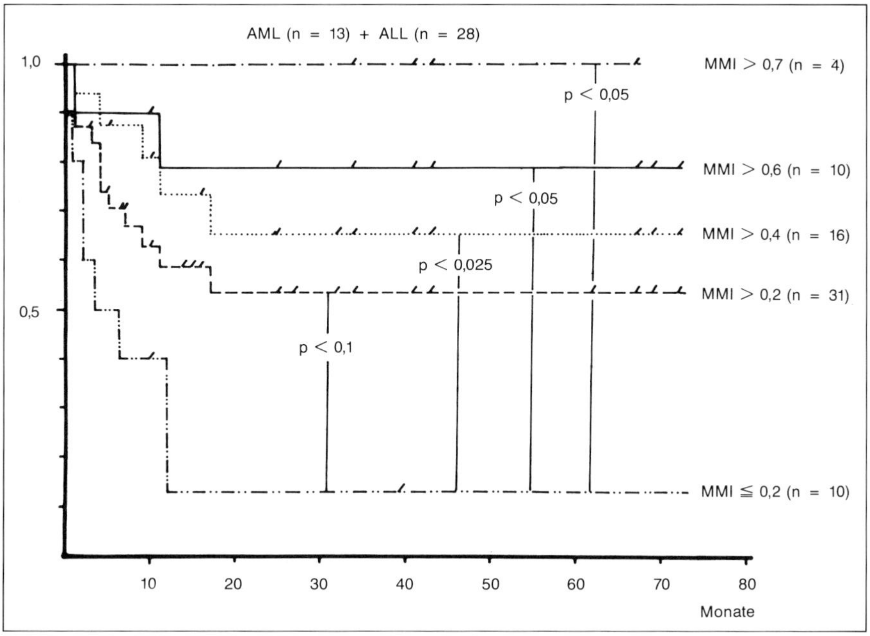

a

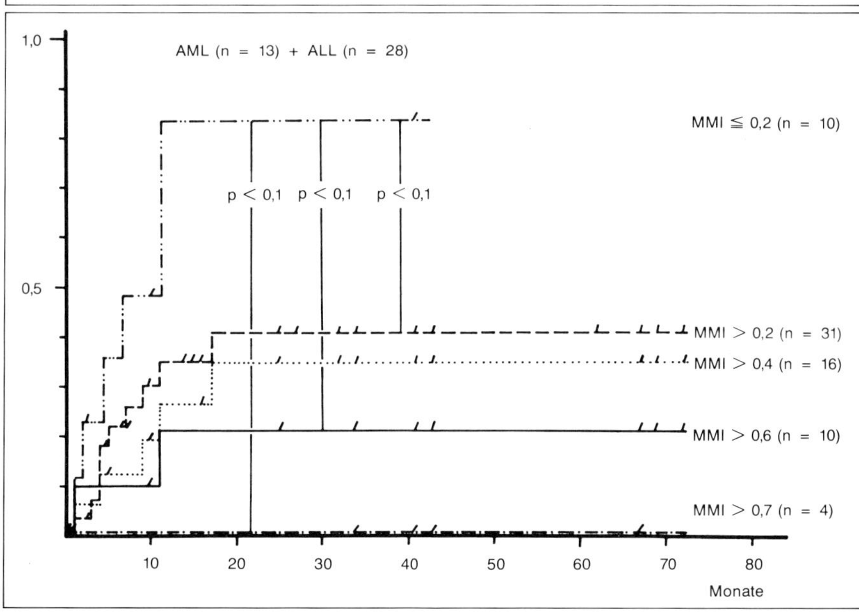

b

Abb. 7. Wahrscheinlichkeit des *a)* DFS und *b)* Rezidives nach AKMT in Abhängigkeit vom myeloischen Mitose-Index (MMI) bei ALL plus AML (KMT-Gruppe Leipzig).

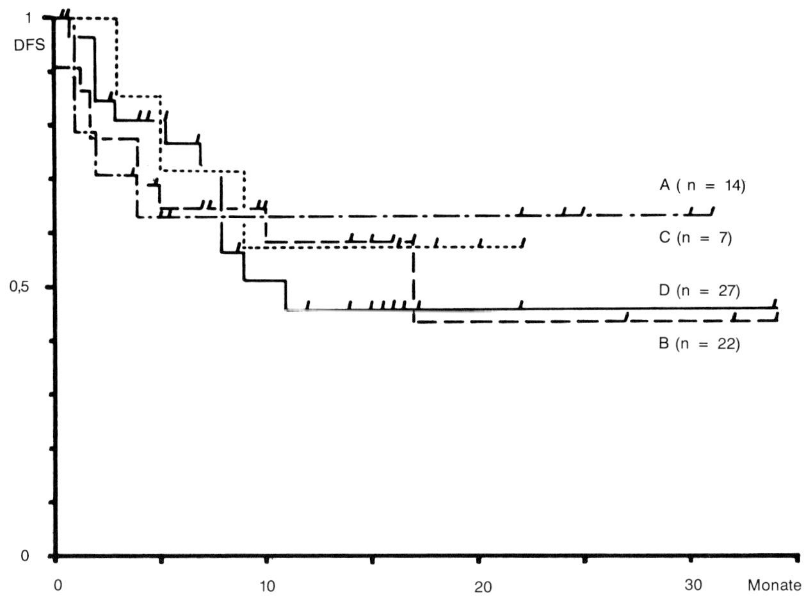

Abb. 8. Zwischenauswertung der Postremissionstherapie von Patienten mit ALL und AML bis 40 Jahre (KMT-Gruppe Leipzig). A = KMT; B = AKMT; C = Doppelkonsolidierung: 6 statt 3 Zyklen, aber keine Erhaltungstherapie; D = monatliche Erhaltungstherapie über 2 Jahre.

Da die prinzipiellen, vor allem aber die praxisrelevanten Möglichkeiten zur Erkennung von Restleukämiezellen derzeitig noch stark begrenzt sind (Tab. 5), fällt die Qualitätsbeurteilung der CR in Mark- und peripheren Stammzellkonzentraten wie auch die laborative Einschätzung der «purging»-Effizienz schwer. Angeregt durch Mitoseuntersuchungen bei Leukämien untersuchten wir 1986 die Mitose-Indices im Autotransplantat und fanden einen Trend zu wenigeren Rezidiven bzw. einer höheren DFS-Wahrscheinlichkeit bei höherem Mitose-Index. Die neuerliche Berechnung an nunmehr 48 Patienten bekräftigte für das DFS diese Vermutung (Abb. 6), nicht jedoch für die Rezidivwahrscheinlichkeit. Werden nur granulierte Mitosen gezählt (myeloischer Mitose-Index), werden diese vorläufigen Befunde gestützt (Abb. 7), die jedoch an einem größeren Material, auch nach konventioneller Therapie, bestätigt werden müssen.

Nachdem vielfältige Studien zur Induktions- und Postremissionstherapie, wie z.B. die von Hoelzer et al. [14] für die ALL und die durch Büchner et al. [2] für die AML, neue Ergebnisse zur remissionserhaltenden Therapie vorlegen konnten, wird die Wertigkeitsbeurteilung der AKMT immer dringlicher, so daß in einigen Ländern bzw. Gruppen mit entsprechend ausgelegten klinisch-kontrollierten Studien begonnen wurde [25]. Die von uns koordinierte multizentrische DDR-Studie erbrachte bei einer früheren Zwischenauswertung der Erwachsenen bis 40 Jahre (aufgrund der kleinen Fallzahlen wurden ALL und AML zusammengefaßt) für die Therapiearme «KMT», «AKMT», «Doppelkonsolidierung ohne Erhaltungstherapie» und «Erhaltungstherapie» bisher keine signifikanten Differenzen (Abb. 8). Vor allem unterscheidet sich bisher die AKMT mit ungepurgtem Mark nicht von der Erhaltungstherapie.

Neben den in unserer Studie implizierten Fragen wären Vergleiche zur «purging»-Effektivität [11, 16] und zum Vergleich der AKMT gegenüber der haplo-identen KMT mit ein- und mehreren Antigen-Differenzen wichtig, künftig wahrscheinlich auch ein Vergleich zur phänotypisch identischen Fremdspender-KMT. Viele Entwicklungen kreuzen sich scheinbar und werfen immer neue Fragen auf, die durch gut koordinierte nationale, besser durch internationale Studien zeitlich angemessen beantwortet werden könnten.

Literatur

1 Anderson, C.C.; Goldstone, A.H.; Linch, D.C.; Jones, H.M.; Franklin, I.M.; Boughton, B.J.; Cawley, J.C.; Richards, J.D.M.: Autologous bone marrow transplantation for patients with acute myeloid leukaemia and acute lymphoblastic leukaemia – a comparison. Bone Marrow Transplant. *1:* 271–279 (1987).

2 Büchner, Th.; Urbanitz, D.; Hiddemann, W.; Koch, P.; Pielken, H.-J.; Kuse, R.; Mohr, A.; Maschmeyer, G.; Kreutzmann, H.; Wendt, F.; Straif, K.; Vaupel, H.A.; Aul, C.; Fischer, J.; Schneider, W.; König, H.J.; Demling, L. Walter, M.; Ludwig, W.D.; Rühl, H.; Seibt, H.; Anders, Ch.; Nowrousian, M.R.; Gassmann, W.; Löffler, H.; Zeile, G.; Hossfeld, D.; von Paleske, A.; Pees, H.W.; Schwamborn, J.; Meusers, P.; Overkamp, F.; Hellriegel, K.-P.; Fülle, H.H.; Bartels, H.; Emmerich, B.; Lengfelder, E.; Donhuijsen-Ant, R.; Ho, A.; Mainzer, K.; Bonfert, B.; Köppler, H.; Thiel, E.; Middelhoff, G.; Nowicki, L.; Zurborn, K.-H.; Siegert, W.; Planker, M.; Augener, W.; Heinecke, A.: Akute myeloische Leukämie (AML) des Erwachsenen. Weiterentwicklung der Therapie auf der Basis klinischer Phase-II- und Phase-III-Studien. Onkologie *9:* 83–91 (1986).

3 Burnett, A.K.: Use of autologous bone marrow transplantation in acute myeloid leukaemia; in Neth, Gallo, Greaves, Kabisch, Modern trends in Human Leukemia VII; Haematology and Blood Transfusion, No. 31, S. 62–66 (Springer, Berlin, Heidelberg, New York 1987).

4 Cahn, J.Y.; Hervé, P.; Flesch, M.; Plouvier, E.; Noir, A.; Racadot, E.; Montcuquet, P.; Behar, C.; Pignon, B.; Boilletot, A.; Lutz, P.; Henon, P.; Rozenbaum, A.; Peters, A.; des Floris, R.L.: Autologous bone marrow transplantation (ABMT) for acute leukaemia in complete remission. Br. J. Haemat. *63:* 457–470 (1986).

5 Carella, A.M.; Martinengo, M.; Santini, G.; Cerri, R.; Congiu, A.; Nati, S.; Gaozza, E.; Giordano, D.; Rossi, E.; Damasio, E.; Risso, M.; Raffo, M.R.; Pungolino, E.; Carlier, P.; D'Amico, T.; Marmont, A.M.: Autologous unpurged bone marrow transplantation for acute non-lymphoblastic leukaemia in first complete remission. Bone Marrow Transplant. *3:* Suppl. 1, S. 73–74 (1988).

6 De Fabritiis, P.; Pulsoni, A.; Sandrelli, A.; Simone, F.; Amadori, S.; Meloni, G.; Mandelli, F.: Efficacy of a combined treatment with ASTA-Z 7654 and VP 16–213 in vitro in eradicating clonogenic tumor cells from human bone marrow. Bone Marrow Transplant. *2:* 287–298 (1987).

7 Gee, A.P.; Boyle, M.D.P.: Purging tumor cells from bone marrow by use of antibody and complement: a critical appraisal. J. Natl. Cancer Inst. *80:* 154–159 (1988).

8 Gorin, N.C.; Douay, L.; Laporte, J.P.; Lopez, M.; Mary, J.Y.; Najman, A.; Salmon, C.; Aegerter, P.; Stachowiak, J.; David, R.; Pene, F.; Kantor, G.; Deloux, J.; Duhamel, E.; van den Akker, J.; Gerota, J.; Parlier, Y.; Duhamel, G.: Autologous bone marrow transplantation using marrow incubated with ASTA Z 7557 in adult acute leukemia. Blood *67:* 1367–1376 (1988).

9 Gorin, N.C.; Aegerter, P.: Autologous bone marrow transplantation for acute leukaemia in remission: Third European survey: March 1986. Bone Marrow Transplant. *1:* Suppl. 1, S. 255–258 (1986).

10 Gorin, N.C.; Aegerter, P.: Autologous bone marrow transplantation for acute leukaemia in remission: 4th EBMTG survey. Bone Marrow Transplant. *2:* Suppl. 1, S. 320–323 (1987).

11 Gorin, N.C.; Aegerter, P.; Auvert, B. for the EBMTG: Autologous bone marrow transplantation (ABMT) for acute leukaemia in remission: fifth European survey. Evidence in favour of marrow purging. Influence of pretansplant intervals. Bone Marrow Transplant. *3:* Suppl. 1, S. 39–47 (1988).

12 Hervé, P.; Flesch, M.; Plouvier, E.; Cahn, J.Y.; Boilletot, A.; Lutz, P.; Munzer, M.; Hénon, Ph.: Autologous bone marrow transplantation in 64 acute leukaemia patients in remission: the Eastern Group experience. An update. Bone Marrow Transplant. *3:* Suppl. 1, S. 54–55 (1988).

13 Hirn, J.; Maraninchi, D.; Delaage, M.; Novakovitsch, G.; Mawas, C.; Hirn, M.; Brailly, H.; Mannoni, P.; Michael, G.; Gastaut, J.A.; Carcassonne, Y.: Autologous BMT after in vitro purging with floating immunobeads. Bone Marrow Transplant. *3:* Suppl. 1, S. 99 (1988).

14 Hoelzer, D.; Thiel, E.; Löffler, H.; Büchner, T.; Ganser, A.; Heil, G.; Koch, P.; Freund, M.; Diedrich, H.; Rühl, H.; Maschmeyer, G.; Lipp, T.; Nowrousian, M.R.; Burkert, M.; Gerecke, D.; Pralle, H.; Müller, U.; Lunscken, Ch.; Fülle, H.; Ho, A.D.; Lüchler, R.; Busch, F.W. Schneider, W.; Görg, Ch.; Emmerich, B.; Braumann, D.; Vaupel, H.A,; von Paleske, A.; Bartels, H.; Neiss, A.; Messerer, D.: Prognostic factors in a multicenter study for treatment of acute lymphoblastic leukemia in adults. Blood *71:* 123–131 (1988).

15 Janossy, G.: Bone marrow purging, Immunol. Today *8:* 253–255 (1987).

16 Janossy, G.; Campana, D.; Amlot, P.: Monoclonal antibodies for autologous BMT (ABMT). Bone Marrow Transplant. *2:* Suppl. 2, S. 66–73 (1987).

17 Körbling, M.; Baumann, M.; Holdermann, E.; Haas, R.; Pezzutto, A.; König, A.; Hunstein, W.; Rother, K.: Autologous blood stem cell transplantation (ABSCT) in 34 patients: its methodological advantage and limitation. Bone Marrow Transplant. *3:* Suppl. 1, S. 51–53 (1988).

18 Körbling, M.; Haas, R.; Baumann, M.; Holdermann, E.; Pezzutto, A.; Mende, U.; König, A.; Rother, K.; Hunstein, W.: A median two year follow-up evaluation of 42 patients with acute leukaemia following ABMT: a single study experience. Bone Marrow Transplant. *3:* Suppl. 1, S. 76–77 (1988).

19 Lotzová, E.: Possible application of natural killer cells and Interleukin-2 in therapy of human leukemia; in Cellular Immunotherapy of Cancer, pp. 259–266 (Alan R. Liss, New York 1987).

20 Mangoni, L.; Degliamtoni, G.; Porcellini, A.; Carella, A.M.; Alessandrino, E.P.; Aglietta, M.; Resegotti, L.; Torlontano, G.; Coleselli, P.; Mozzana, R.; Madon, E.; Rizzoli, V.: Autologous bone marrow transplantation in acute leukemia. Acta haemat. *78:* Suppl. 1, S. 190–193 (1987).

21 Meloni, G.; De Fabritiis, P.; Pulsoni, A.; Sandrelli, A.; Giarnieri, V.; Moleti, M.L.; Mandelli, F.: Autologous bone marrow transplantation in children with haematological malignancies. Bone Marrow Transplant. *3:* Suppl. 1, S. 103 (1988).

22 Meloni, G.; De Fabritiis, P.; Pulsoni, A.; Giarnier, V.; Petti, M.C.; Amadori, S.; Mandelli, F.: BAVC conditioning regimen and ABMT in patients with acute myelogenous leukaemia (AML) in second complete remission (CR). Bone Marrow Transplant. *3:* Suppl. 1, S. 72 (1988).

23 Nustad, K.; Michaelsen, T.E.; Kierulf, B.; Fjeld, J.G.; Kvalheim, G.; Pihl, A.; Ugelstadt, J.; Funderud, S.: Antigen binding properties of antibodies coated on magnetic polymer beads. Bone Marrow Transplant. *2:* Suppl. 2, S. 81–83 (1987).

24 Okamoto, S.; Olson, A.C.; Vogler, W.R.; Winton, E.F.: Purging leukemic cells from simulated human remission marrow with Alkyl-Lysophospholipid. Blood *69:* 1381–1387 (1987).

25 Proctor, S.J.; Hamilton, P.J.; Taylor, P.; Carey, P.; Hargrave, S.; Evans, R.G.B.; Summerfield, G.; Finney, R.; Saunders, P.; Goff, D.; Reid, M.M.: A comparative study of combination chemotherapy versus marrow transplant in first remission in adult acute lymphoblastic leukaemia. Br. J. Haemat. *69:* 35–39 (1988).

26 Ramsay, N.; LeBien, T.; Nesbit, M.; McGlave, Ph.; Weisdorf, D.; Kenyon, P.; Hurd, D.; Goldman, A.; Kim, T.; Kersey, J.: Autologous bone marrow transplantation for patients with acute lymphoblastic leukemia in second or subsequent remission: results of bone marrow treated with monoclonal antibodies VA-1, BA-2, and BA-3 plus complement. Blood *66:* 508–513 (1985).

27 Santos, G.W.; Tutschka, P.J.; Brookmeyer, R.; Saral, R.; Beschorner, W.E.; Bias, W.B.; Braine, H.G.; Burns, W.H.; Elfenbein, G.J.; Kaizer, H.; Mellits, D.; Sensenbrenner, L.L.; Stuart, R.K.; Yeager, A.M.: Marrow transplantation for acute nonlymphocytic leukemia after treatment with busulfan and cyclophosphamide. New Engl. J. Med. *309:* 1347–1353 (1983).

28 Santos, G.W.; Saral, R.; Burns, W.H.; braine, H.G.; Sensenbrenner, L.L.; Wingard, J.R.; Yeager, A.M.; Jones, R.; Ambinder, R.F.; Rowley, S.D.; May, S.; Vogelsang, B.G.: Allogeneic, syngeneic and autologous marrow transplantation in the acute leukemias and lymphomas – Baltimore experiences. Acta haemat. *78:* Suppl. 1, S. 175–180 (1987).

29 Siever, F.: Marrow purging by merocyanine 540-mediatd photolysis. Bone Marrow Transplant. *2:* Suppl. 2, S. 29–33 (1987).

30 Simonsson, B.; Burnett, A.K.; Hann, I.; Prentice, H.G.; Gibson, B.; Lönnerholm, G.; Smedmyr, B.; Morrison, A.; Todd, A.; Tötterman, Th.; Öberg, G.; Campana, D.; Janossy, G.: Myeloablative therapy with monoclonal antibody purged marrow rescue in high-risk acute lymphoblastic leukaemia. Bone Marrow Transplant. *3:* Suppl. 1, pp. 75 (1988).

31 Stewart, P.; Buckner, C.D.; Bensinger, W.; Appelbaum, F.; Fefer, A.; Clift, R.; Storb, R.; Sanders, J.; Meyers, J.; Hill, R.; Thomas, E.D.: Autologous marrow transplantation in patients with acute nonlymphocytic leukemia in first remission. Exp. Hematol. *13:* 267–272 (1985).

32 Teichmann, J.V.; Ludwig, W.-D.; Seibt-Jung, H.; Sieber, G.; Thiel, E.: Induction of lymphokine-aktivated killer (LAK) cells against human leukemia cells; in Neth, Gallo, Greaves, Kabisch, Modern trends in Human Leukemia VIII, Wilsede 1988 (im Druck).

33 To, L.B.; Juttner, C.A.: Annotation: Peripheral blood stem cell autografting. A new therapeutic option for AML? Br. J. Haemat. *66:* 285–288 (1987).

34 Verdonck, L.F.; Dekker, A.W.; Vendrik, P.J.; van Kempen, M.L.; Schornagel, J.H.; Rozenberg-Arska, M.; deGast, C.: Intensive cytoreductive therapy followed by autologous bone marrow transplantation for patients with hematologic malignancies or solid tumors. Cancer *60:* 289–295 (1987).

35 Yeager, A.M.; Wiley, J.M.; Jones, R.; Rowley, S.D.; Zuehsdorf, M.; Colvin, O.M.; Santos, G.W.: Pharmacologic treatment of bone marrow to eliminate clonogenic tumor cells: laboratory and clinical studies. Bone Marrow Transplant. *2:* Suppl. 2, pp. 34–38 (1987).

Prof. Dr. sc. med. W. Helbig, Karl-Marx-Universität Leipzig, Klinik für Innere Medizin, Johannisallee 32, DDR-7010 Leipzig

Beitr Onkol, vol. 36, pp. 35–43 (Karger, Basel 1989)

Allogene Knochenmarktransplantation bei akuten Leukämien

N. Schmitz, W. Gassmann, H. Löffler

II. Medizinische Klinik und Poliklinik der Christian-Albrechts-Universität Kiel

Einleitung

Die erste allogene Knochenmarktransplantation (KMT) bei einem Patienten mit akuter Leukämie ist von Thomas et al. in Seattle durchgeführt worden. Er berichtete 1959 über erste klinische Erfahrungen mit dieser neuen Methode [1]. Nach einer Vorbehandlung, die zunächst nur aus einer Ganzkörperbestrahlung mit 1000 rad bestand, erhielten Patienten mit therapierefraktären Lymphomen oder Leukämien Leichenknochenmark oder Knochenmark eines freiwilligen Lebendspenders. Das HLA-System war zu dieser Zeit noch unbekannt, eine Testung der Gewebeverträglichkeit zwischen Knochenmarkempfänger und -spender demzufolge nicht möglich. Entsprechend dieser äußerst ungünstigen Ausgangssituation waren auch die Ergebnisse der allogenen Knochenmarktransplantation miserabel. Patienten, die nicht bereits in den ersten Wochen nach Transplantation an den Folgen einer Transplantat-Abstoßung oder einer Transplantat-gegen-Wirt-Reaktion («graft-versus-host-disease», GVHD) verstarben, erlitten sehr bald ein leukämisches Rezidiv.

Einen entscheidenden Durchbruch für die allogene Knochenmarktransplantation stellte die Entdeckung des HLA-Systems in seiner Bedeutung für die klinische Knochenmarktransplantation dar. Nach Beschränkung auf Patienten mit einem HLA-identischen Geschwister konnte die Abstoßungsrate bei Leukämiepatienten dramatisch gesenkt werden, der Prozentsatz von Abstoßungen liegt heute bei etwa 1% [2]. Auch die Inzidenz und Schwere der GVHD konnte verringert werden; trotzdem bleibt die GVHD auch heute eine ernstzunehmende Komplikation der allogenen Knochenmarktransplantation. Dies gilt insbesondere deshalb, weil sie in hohem

Maße mit dem Auftreten einer interstitiellen Pneumonie korreliert, die die heute schwerwiegendste Komplikation der allogenen Knochenmarktransplantation überhaupt darstellt.

Nach Einführung einer kombinierten Chemo-/Radiotherapie vor Knochenmarktransplantation konnte die Rezidivrate gesenkt werden, es gelang erstmals, einige wenige Patienten auch in fortgeschrittenen Stadien von akuten Leukämien langfristig am Leben zu erhalten, ohne daß ein Rezidiv auftrat. Durch Vorverlegung des Transplantationstermins in die erste Remission konnten die Ergebnisse weiter verbessert werden, nichtsdestoweniger sind bei einer augenblicklichen Rezidivrate von etwa 20% auch für früh transplantierte Patienten Verbesserungen wünschenswert. Dies gilt in verstärktem Maße für Patienten, die in später Remission oder im Rezidiv transplantiert werden müssen.

Neben den bereits erwähnten klinischen Problemen GVHD, interstitielle Pneumonie und Leukämierezidiv stellt die Beschränkung auf Patienten mit HLA-identem Geschwister selbstverständlich eine entscheidende Limitation der Knochenmarktransplantation dar. Empirischen Untersuchungen zufolge kann höchstens jeder dritte Patient, für den von seiten seiner Erkrankung die allogene Knochenmarktransplantation eine optimale Therapieform darstellen würde, tatsächlich damit rechnen, daß ein kompatibler Spender innerhalb der Familie gefunden wird und eine Transplantation durchgeführt werden kann.

Im folgenden soll zu den oben geschilderten Problemen der Knochenmarktransplantation Stellung genommen und der aktuelle Stand diskutiert werden. Eigene Untersuchungen mit einem neuen Konditionierungsprotokoll, das hohe antileukämische Wirkung entfaltet, werden vorgestellt.

Transplantat-gegen-Wirt-Reaktion (GVHD)

Auch bei einer Altersbeschränkung auf Patienten unter 50 Jahre und solche Patienten, die ein HLA-kompatibles Geschwister besitzen, müssen 40–50% aller Transplantationspatienten mit dem Auftreten einer GVHD rechnen. Schwere Formen der GVHD mit Exanthem, Diarrhoe und Ikterus betreffen etwa ein Drittel aller Patienten mit GVHD oder 20% aller allogen transplantierten Patienten. Transplantat-gegen-Wirt-Reaktionen der Grade III und IV sind lebensbedrohlich, da die zur Behandlung notwendigen hohen und höchsten Dosen von Immunsuppressiva eine ausgeprägte Infektneigung bewirken. Häufigste Todesursache im Rahmen einer schweren

GVHD sind deshalb Infektionen viraler, mykotischer oder bakterieller Genese. Nachdem zunächst eine GVHD-Prophylaxe in Form einer Monotherapie mit Methotrexat beziehungsweise Cyclosporin A üblich war, haben Kombinationen mehrerer Immunsuppressiva beispielsweise von Cyclosporin A und Prednisolon oder Cyclosporin A und Methotrexat gewisse Fortschritte gebracht [4, 5]. Insgesamt sind die medikamentösen Versuche zur Unterdrückung der GVHD jedoch weiterhin nicht befriedigend.

Mit Hilfe einer In-vitro-T-Zell-Depletion des Spenderknochenmarkes kann die GVHD verhindert werden [6]. Leider ist eine effektive T-Zell-Depletion immer mit einem erhöhten Abstoßungsrisiko und zumindest bei einigen Leukämien auch mit einem höheren Rezidivrisiko verbunden [7]. Aus diesem Grunde ist das Überleben von Patienten, die T-Zell-depletiertes Knochenmark erhalten haben, bisher nicht besser als nach der Übertragung unmanipulierten Knochenmarks. Erst wenn Möglichkeiten gefunden werden können, Abstoßungsrate und Rezidivquote nach Transplantation T-Zell-depletierten Knochenmarks zu senken, wird dieses Verfahren breiteren Eingang in die Klinik finden können.

Weitere Forschung auf diesem Gebiet ist dringend notwendig, wenn mehr Patienten von der Methode der allogenen Transplantation profitieren sollen.

Interstitielle Pneumonie

Die interstitielle Pneumonie stellt heute die schwerwiegendste Komplikation der allogenen Knochenmarktransplantation dar. Nach einer Erhebung der International Bone Marrow Transplant Registry (IBMTR) beträgt die aktuarielle Inzidenz interstitieller Pneumonien 35±4%; etwa 80% aller Patienten, die an einer interstitiellen Pneumonie erkranken, versterben an dieser Komplikation [8]. Die Erkrankung wird in über 50% der Patienten durch Zytomegalieviren verursacht, die entweder zum Zeitpunkt der Transplantation latent bereits vorhanden sind oder mit dem Spenderknochenmark oder anderen im Posttransplantationsverlauf notwendigen Blutprodukten übertragen werden. Die Erkrankung tritt oftmals während einer schweren akuten GVHD auf; überraschend war, daß bei einer Untersuchung der Todesursachen von 196 CML-Patienten in mehr als 50% der letal verlaufenden interstitiellen Pneumonien keine, beziehungsweise lediglich eine milde GVHD vorhanden war [9].

Bei CMV-negativen Patienten, die Knochenmark von einem CMV-negativen Geschwister erhalten, läßt sich die Inzidenz CMV-assoziierter interstitieller Pneumonien durch ausschließliche Verwendung von CMV-negativen Blutprodukten dramatisch senken. Bei CMV-positiven Knochenmarkempfängern sind diese Maßnahmen allenfalls von fraglichem Wert.

Wegen der vielen Parameter, die das Ergebnis beeinflussen können, steht der schlüssige Beweis der Wirksamkeit eines CMV-Hyperimmunglobulins zur Prophylaxe der CMV-assoziierten interstitiellen Pneumonie letztendlich aus, mehrere Studien legen einen positiven Effekt solcher Hyperimmunglobuline jedoch nahe [10–12]. Interessant ist die Beobachtung, daß auch die prophylaktische Gabe von Aciclovir eine statistisch signifikante Senkung der Inzidenz von interstitiellen Pneumonien bewirken soll [13].

Die Therapie der CMV-assoziierten interstitiellen Pneumonie ist unbefriedigend, höchste Dosen von CMV-Hyperimmunglobulin sind den Beweis ihrer Wirksamkeit bisher schuldig geblieben, auch die alleinige Gabe von Ganciclovir, das in vitro sowie bei anderen Organmanifestationen der CMV-Infektionen durchaus wirksam ist, hat enttäuscht [14]. Ob die kombinierte Behandlung mit Hyperimmunglobulin und Ganciclovir die Ergebnisse verbessern kann, muß offenbleiben.

Neben dem Zytomegalievirus sind in selteneren Fällen andere Viren der Herpesgruppe, Pilze oder Pneumocystis carinii Ursache einer interstitiellen Pneumonie. Eine aggressive Diagnostik und Therapie können in diesen Fällen lebensrettend sein.

Bei etwa einem Drittel aller interstitiellen Pneumonien findet sich trotz intensiver Suche nach einem Erreger kein Hinweis für die infektiöse Genese. Diese als idiopathische interstitielle Pneumonien bezeichnete Gruppe bietet kaum therapeutische Möglichkeiten.

Rezidive nach allogener Knochenmarktransplantation

Die Rezidivhäufigkeit und das Überleben nach allogener Knochenmarktransplantation für Patienten mit akuten Leukämien ist in Tabelle 1 in Abhängigkeit vom Krankheitsstadium aufgelistet. Die Zahlen entsprechen den Erfahrungen an großen Patientenkollektiven, wie sie von der IBMTR und der European Bone Marrow Transplantation Group (EBMT) publiziert worden sind. Die aufgelisteten Rezidivraten beziehen sich im wesentlichen auf Patienten, die eine Vorbehandlung mit Cyclophosphamid (120 mg/kg Körpergewicht) und Ganzkörperbestrahlung (9–12 Gy) erhalten haben. Insbesondere in fortgeschrittenen Stadien sind die Rezidivquoten erschreckend hoch, so daß ein verbesserter antileukämischer Effekt des Kon-

Tabelle 1. Rezidivquote und krankheitsfreies Überleben nach allogener KMT

	Rezidive	Überleben
AML, 1. Remission	20%	50%
AML, 2. Remission	40%	30%
ALL, 1. Remission	25%	45%
ALL,, 2. Remission*	40–50%	20–30%
AML/ALL, fortgeschrittene Stadien	50–75%	10–30%
CML, chronische Phase	15%	50%

* Rezidivquote und krankheitsfreies Überleben sind abhängig davon, ob bei Diagnose bestimmte Risikofaktoren vorlagen

ditionierungsprotokolls dringend erwünscht ist. Trotz einer Vielzahl von Versuchen, die antileukämische Potenz des Konditionierungsprotokolls zu steigern, ist auf diesem Gebiet bis in die letzten Jahre hinein kein entscheidender Fortschritt erzielt worden. In vielen Fällen wurde der Vorteil eines besseren Effektes auf die Leukämie durch eine höhere Toxizität des neuen Behandlungsprotokolls egalisiert.

In den letzten Jahren sind einige neue Konditionierungsprotokolle entwickelt worden, die bei möglicherweise besserer antileukämischer Wirkung keine wesentliche Toxizitätssteigerung aufweisen. In dieser Hinsicht sind insbesondere die Kombination hyperfraktionierter Ganzkörperbestrahlung und Cyclophosphamid [15], Busulfan und Cyclophosphamid [16, 17] sowie die Kombination von Ganzkörperbestrahlung und hochdosiertem Cytosin-Arabinosid [18] beziehungsweise hochdosiertem VP 16 [19, 20] erwähnenswert. Die Kombination fraktionierte Ganzkörperbestrahlung und hochdosiertes Etoposid (60–70 mg/kg Körpergewicht) ist in Kiel experimentell und klinisch geprüft worden [20, 21]. Das krankheitsfreie Überleben von 33 Patienten mit akuten Leukämien – meist in weit fortgeschrittenen Stadien – lag nach einer Beobachtungszeit von 6–35 Monaten (Median 18 Monate) bei 56,6%, die Rezidivquote betrug 11,9%. Eine neuere Auswertung unserer Daten zeigt, daß dieses Konditionierungsprotokoll insbesondere bei Patienten mit akuter lymphatischer Leukämie effektiv und gut verträglich ist. Das krankheitsfreie Überleben und die aktuarielle Rezidivrate für 20 in Kiel transplantierte Patienten mit akuter lymphatischer Leukämie sind in Abbildung 1 dargestellt. Vorläufige Ergebnisse mit diesem Protokoll in der gesamten Bundesrepublik scheinen diesen Trend zu bestätigen.

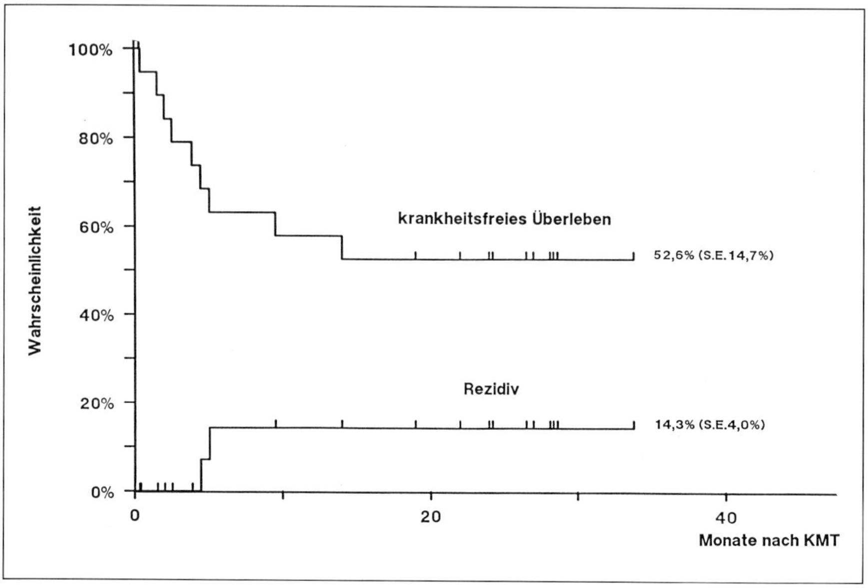

Abb. 1. Krankheitsfreies Überleben und kumulative Rezidivwahrscheinlichkeit bei 20 Patienten mit ALL in verschiedenen Stadien.

Spenderauswahl

Die Beschränkung der allogenen Knochenmarktransplantation auf Patienten unter 50 Jahre, die einen HLA-kompatiblen Spender in der Familie haben, stellt eine erhebliche Einschränkung der Anwendbarkeit des Verfahrens dar. Die Anhebung der Altergrenze scheint solange unrealistisch, wie eine wirksamere Bekämpfung der GVHD aussteht. Inzidenz und Schwere der GVHD nehmen mit jeder Lebensdekade zu, so daß Patienten über 45 Jahren nur in Einzelfällen transplantiert werden sollten.

Für Patienten ohne genotypisch identische Spender gelingt es gelegentlich, in der erweiterten Familie einen phänotypisch identischen Spender zu finden. Bis auf diese seltenen Ausnahmen sind die Erfahrungen mit allogener Knochenmarktransplantation von teilkompatiblen Familienspendern enttäuschend [22]. Nur solchen Patienten, die eine extrem schlechte Prognose aufweisen, sollte eine allogene Knochenmarktransplantation von einem Familienspender angeboten werden, der in ein oder höchstens zwei Loci des HLA-Systems differiert.

Durch Aufbau von Fremdspenderkarteien in England, den USA und ansatzweise auch in der Bundesrepublik Deutschland, besteht mittlerweile die Möglichkeit, für einige Patienten ohne Familienspender einen HLA-vollidentischen Fremdspender ausfindig zu machen. Das Verfahren ist bisher sehr langwierig, so daß zwischen Beginn der Spendersuche und Abschluß oft Monate vergehen. Solche Zeiträume sind für Patienten mit akuten Leukämien inakzeptabel, da die Natur der Erkrankung solche Zeitverzögerungen nicht erlaubt. Weil die Ergebnisse der allogenen Knochenmarktransplantation von HLA-vollidentischen Fremdspendern bisher jedoch sehr ermutigend sind [23], wird man durch eine verbesserte Logistik eine schnellere Spendersuche anstreben müssen. Es bleibt abzuwarten, ob bei Patienten mit akuten Leukämien ähnlich gute Ergebnisse erzielt werden können wie das bei CML-Patienten der Fall ist.

Literatur

1 Thomas, E.D.; Lochte, H.L.; Ferrebee, J.W.: Irradiation of the entire body and marrow transplantation: Some observations and comments. Blood *14:* 1–23 (1959).

2 Beatty, P.G.; Clift, R.A.; Mickelson, E.M.; Nisperos, B.B.; Flournoy, N.; Martin, P.J.; Sanders, J.E.; Stewart, P.; Buckner, C.D.; Storb, R.; Thomas, E.D.; Hansen, J.A.: Marrow transplantation from related donors other than HLA-identical siblings. New Engl. J. Med. *313:* 765–771 (1985).

3 Gale, R.P.; Bortin, M.M.; Van Bekkum, D.W.; Biggs, J.C.; Dicke, K.A.; Gluckman, E.; Good, R.A.; Hoffmann, R.G.; Kay, H.E.M.; Kersey, J.H.; Marmont, A.; Masaoka, T.; Rimm, A.A.; Van Rood, J.J.; Zwaan, F.E.: Risk factors for acute graft-versus-host disease. Br. J. Haematol. *67:* 397–406 (1987).

4 Forman, S.J.; Blume, K.G.; Krance, R.A.; Miner, P.J.; Metter, G.E.; Hill, L.R.; O'Donnell, M.R.; Nademanee, A.P.; Snyder, D.S.: A prospective randomized study of acute graft-v-host disease in 107 patients with leukemia: methotrexate/prednisone v. cyclosporine A/prednisone. Transplant. Proc. *19:* 2605–2607 (1987).

5 Storb, R.; Deeg, H.J.; Whitehead, J.; Appelbaum, F.; Beatty, P.; Bensinger, W.; Buckner, C.D.; Clift, R.; Doney, K.; Farewell, V.; Hansen, J.; Hill, R.; Lum, L.; Martin, P.; McGuffin, R.; Sanders, J.; Stewart, P.; Sullivan, K.; Witherspoon, R.; Yee, G.; Thomas, E.D.: Methotrexate and cyclosporine compared with cyclosporine alone for prophylaxis of acute graft versus host disease after marrow transplantation for leukemia. New Engl. J. Med. *314:* 729–735 (1986).

6 Waldmann, H.; Polliak, A.; Hale, G. et al.: Elimination of graft-versus-host disease by in-vitro depletion of alloreactive lymohocytes with a monoclonal rat antibody (Campath-1). Lancet *ii:* 483–486 (1984).

7 Goldman, J.M.; Gale, R.P.; Horowitz, M.M.; Biggs, J.C.; Champlin, R.E.; Gluckman, E.; Hoffmann, R. G.; Jacobsen, S.J.; Marmont, A.M.; McGlave, P.B.; Messner, H.A.; Rimm, A.A.; Rozman, C.; Speck, B.; Tura, S.; Weiner, R.S.; Bortin, M.M.: Bone marrow

transplantation for chronic leukemia in chronic phase. Ann. Intern. Med. *108:* 806–814 (1988).

8 Weiner, R.S.; Bortin, M.M.; Gale, R.P.; Gluckman, E.; Kay, H.E.M.; Kolb, H.-J.; Hartz, A.J.; Rimm, A.A.: Interstitial pneumonitis following bone marrow transplantation: assessment of risk factors. Ann Intern. Med. *104:* 168 (1986).

9 Löffler, H.; Schmitz, N.: Allogeneic bone marrow transplantation for CML in Austria and West Germany. Blut *57:* 221 (1988).

10 Kubanek, B.; Ernst, P.; Ostendorf, P.; Schafer, U.; Wolf, H.: Preliminary data of a controlled trial of intravenous hyperimmune globulin in the prevention of cytomegalovirus infection in bone marrow transplant recipients. Transplant. Proc. *17:* 468–469 (1985).

11 Winston, D.J.; Pollard, R.B.; Ho, W.G. et al.: Cytomegalovirus immune plasma in bone marrow transplant recipients. Ann. Intern. Med. *97:* 11–18 (1982).

12 Condie, R.M.; O-Reilly, R.J.: Prevention of cytomegalovirus infection by prophylaxis with an intravenous, hyperimmune, native, unmodified cytomegalovirus globulin. Am. J. Med. *76:* 134–141 (1984).

13 Meyers, J.D.; Reed, E.C.; Shepp, D.H.; Thornquist, M.; Dandliker, P.S.; Vigary, C.A.; Flournoy, N.; Kirk, L.E.; Kersey, J.H.; Thomas, E.D.; Balfour, H.H.; Acyclovir for prevention of cytomegalovirus infection and disease after allogeneic marrow transplantation. New Engl. J. Med. *318:* 70–75 (1988).

14 Shepp, D.H.; Dandliker, P.S.; de Miranda, P.; Burnett, T.C.; Cederberg, D.M.; Kirk, L.E.; Mayers, J.D.; Activity of 9-[2-hydroxy-1-(hydroxymethyl)ethoxymethyl]guanine in the treatment of cytomegalovirus pneumonia. Ann. Intern. Med. *103:* 368–373 (1985).

15 Brochstein, J.A.; Kernan, N.A.; Groshen, S.; Cirrincione, C.; Shank, B.; Emanuel, D.; Laver, J.; O'Reilly, R.J.: Allogeneic bone marrow transplantation after hyperfractionated total-body irradiation and cyclophosphamide in children with acute leukemia. New Engl. J. Med. *317:* 1618–1624 (1987).

16 Santos, G.W.; Tutschka, P.J.; Brockmeyer, R.; Saral, R.; Beschorner, W.E.; Bias, W.B.; Braine, H.G.; Burns, W.H.; Elfenbein, G.J.; Kaizer, H.; Mellits, D.; Sensenbrenner, L.L.; Stuart, R.K.; Yeager, A.M.: Marrow transplantation for acute nonlymphocytic leukemia after treatment with busulfan and cyclophosphamide. New Engl. J. Med. *309:* 1347–1353 (1983).

17 Tutschka, P.J.; Copelan, E.A.; Klein, J.P.: Bone marrow transplantation for leukemia following a new busulfan and cyclophosphamide regimen. Blood *70:* 1382–1388 (1987).

18 Coccia, P.F.; Strandjord, S.E.; Warkentin, P.I.; Cheung, N.-K.V.; Gordon, E.M.; Novak, L.J.; Shina, D.C.; Herzig, R.H.: High-dose cytosine arabinoside and fractionated total-body irradiation: an improved preparative regimen for bone marrow transplantation of children with acute lymphoblastic leukemia in remission. Blood *70:* 888–893 (1988).

19 Blume, K.G.; Forman, S.J.; O'Donnell, M.R.; Doroshow, J.H.; Krance, R.A.; Nademanee, A.P.; Snyder, D.S.; Schmidt, G.M.; Fahey, J.L.; Metter, G.E.; Hill, L.R.; Findley, D.O.; Sniecinski, I.J.: Total body irradiation and high-dose etoposide: a new preparatory regimen for bone marrow transplantation in patients with advanced hematologic malignancies. Blood *69:* 1015–1020 (1987).

20 Schmitz, N.; Gassmann, W.; Rister, M.; Johannson, W.; Suttorp, M.; Brix, F.; Holthuis, J.J.M.; Heit, W.; Hertenstein, B.; Schaub, J.; Löffler, H.: Fractionated total body irradiation and high-dose VP 16–213 followed by allogeneic bone marrow transplantation in advanced leukemias. Blood *72:* 1567–1573 (1988).

21 Gassmann, W.; Uharek, L.; Wottge, H.U.; Schmitz, N.; Loeffler, H.; Mueller-Ruchholtz, W.: Comparison of cyclophosphamide, cytarabine and etoposide as immunosuppressive agents before allogeneic bone marrow transplantation. Blood *72:* 1574–1579 (1988).

22 Gingrich, R.D.; Ginder, G.D.; Goeken, N.E.; Howe, C.W.S.; Wen, B.-C.; Hussey, D.H.; Fyfe, M.A.: Allogeneic marrow grafting with partially mismatched, unrelated marrow donors. Blood *71:* 1375–1381 (1988).

23 McGlave, P.; Scott, E.; Ramsay, N.; Arthur, D.; Blazar, B.; McCullough, J.; Kersey, J.: Unrelated donor bone marrow transplantation therapy for chronic myelogenous leukemia. Blood *70:* 877–881 (1987).

N. Schmitz, II. Medizinische Klinik und Poliklinik der Christian-Albrechts-Universität, D-2300 Kiel 1 (BRD)

Beitr Onkol, vol. 36, pp. 44–57 (Karger, Basel 1989)

Grundlagen und neuere Entwicklungen der Therapie der Non-Hodgkin-Lymphome

M. Engelhard, G. Brittinger

Medizinische Universitätsklinik, Essen

Einleitung

Im Gegensatz zu dem eher einheitlichen Krankheitsbild des M. Hodgkin umfaßt der Begriff der Non-Hodgkin-Lymphome (NHL) eine Gruppe klinisch sehr variabel erscheinender Neoplasien lymphatischen Ursprungs, deren enge Verwandtschaft erst durch eine differenzierte immunohistologische Analyse erkannt und genauer definiert werden konnte. Dadurch war dann auch die Grundlage gegeben für prospektive Untersuchungen zur klinischen Symptomatik und therapeutischen Beeinflußbarkeit dieser Erkrankungen. So waren im Rahmen einer multizentrischen Beobachtungsstudie der Kieler Lymphomgruppe von 1975–1980 1127 Patienten mit NHL rekrutiert, nach zentraler histologischer Begutachtung gemäß den Kriterien der Kiel-Klassifikation [22, 34] den einzelnen Entitäten zugeordnet, nach weitgehend einheitlichen Prinzipien behandelt und bis zu 10 Jahren nachbeobachtet worden [4]. Die aus dieser Studie gewonnenen Erkenntnisse haben wesentlich zum Verständnis des klinischen Bildes der verschiedenen Lymphom-Entitäten beigetragen, wobei die Ergebnisse inzwischen durch weitere weltweit gesammelte und zumindest teilweise vergleichbare Erfahrungen unterstützt werden.

Die genauere Datenanalyse ließ folgende allgemeine Merkmale erkennen: Die niedrig-malignen NHL sind gekennzeichnet durch eine geringe Proliferationsrate, die in einem relativ günstigen Spontanverlauf bei oft langjährig fehlender Behandlungsbedürftigkeit zum Ausdruck kommt. Zumindest in den lokalisierten Stadien sind diese Lymphome durch Radiotherapie potentiell heilbar. Liegt jedoch bereits initial ein therapiebedürftiges fortgeschrittenes Stadium vor oder entwickeln sich im Verlauf Symptome, die eine Behandlungsindikation darstellen, z.B. Auftreten einer B-Symptomatik, Progredienz der Lymphome, Entwicklung einer Anämie und/oder Thrombozytopenie, so darf bei Einsatz einer wenig intensiven zytostatischen Chemotherapie (z.B. Chlorambucil, Prednison) ein recht gutes, meist wiederholbares Ansprechen mit Induktion von Teil- oder Vollremissionen erwartet werden. Die erreichten Remissionen erweisen sich jedoch als instabil mit einer anhaltenden und den Verlauf letztlich terminierenden Rezidivneigung, so daß bislang die niedrig-malignen NHL in den fortgeschrittenen Stadien als unheilbar – zumindest durch konventionelle Chemotherapie – angesehen werden müssen.

Die hochmalignen NHL sind dagegen charakterisiert durch eine hohe Proliferationsrate, welche der klinisch zu beobachtenden Tendenz zur raschen Generalisation zugrunde liegt, so daß allgemeine Übereinkunft besteht über die Notwendigkeit des raschen Einsatzes einer intensiven Therapie. Dabei kann alerdings durch die Induktion von Teilremissionen die Prognose kaum verbessert werden, während eine anhaltende Vollremission die Chance der Heilung beinhaltet. Im streng lokalisierten Stadium I (Ann-Arbor-Klassifikation), definiert und abgesichert durch eine invasive Diagnostik, ist bei bestimmten hochmalignen NHL, z.B. den zentroblastischen Lymphomen, die initiale Radiotherapie kurativ wirksam [5].

In den Stadien II–IV, bei allen lymphoblastischen Lymphomen sowie in den Fällen, wo eine genauere Zuordnung des Tumors nicht möglich ist (sog. unklassifizierbare hochmaligne NHL), ist eine stabile Vollremission nur durch den Einsatz einer intensiven Polychemotherapie zu erreichen. Dennoch muß vor allem innerhalb der ersten zwei Jahre nach Abschluß der Induktionstherapie, in geringerem Umfang auch noch später, mit Rezidiven gerechnet werden. Die Prognose dieser Patienten wie auch derjenigen Kranken, die wegen des unzureichenden Ansprechens auf die Induktionstherapie von vornherein als therapierefraktär einzuschätzen sind, ist derzeit noch sehr ungünstig. Nur in Ausnahmefällen gelingt es, durch eine erneute Chemo- und/oder Radiotherapie eine zweite anhaltende Remission zu erreichen [7, 17].

Der klinische Verlauf der NHL wird veranschaulicht durch die Überlebenswahrscheinlichkeitskurven (Abb. 1). Dabei kennzeichnet der kontinuierlich abfallende Kurvenverlauf, der durch die anhaltende, therapeutisch wenig beeinflußbare Rezidivneigung bedingt ist, die niedrig-malignen NHL. Im Gegensatz dazu steht eine nach ein bis zwei Jahren erkennbare Plateaubildung der Kurven der hochmalignen NHL, deren Niveau durch das Kollektiv der geheilten Patienten bestimmt wird. Das individuelle Gefälle der

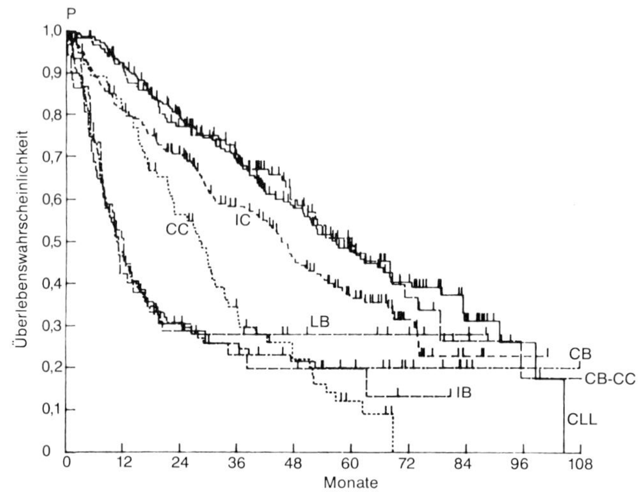

Abb. 1. Überlebenswahrscheinlichkeit der Patienten mit den Hauptentitäten der Non-Hodgkin-Lymphome (entsprechend der Kiel-Klassifikation). Ergebnisse der prospektiven Beobachtungsstudie der Kieler Lymphomgruppe [4]. CLL: chronische lymphatische Leukämie (n = 217); IC: LP-Immunozytom (n = 202); CC: zentrozytisches Lymphom (n = 76); CB-CC: zentroblastisch-zentrozytisches Lymphom (n = 113); CB: zentroblastisches Lymphom (n = 89); IB: immunoblastisches Lymphom (n = 45); LB: lymphoblastisches Lymphom (n = 51). Das niedrige Niveau der Überlebenswahrscheinlichkeit der Patienten mit hochmalignen Lymphomen wird weitgehend durch die wenig intensive Polychemotherapie (vorwiegend COP ± Methotrexat; C-MOPP) erklärt, die während dieser bereits 1975 begonnenen Studie durchgeführt wurde.

für jeden Histologie-Typ charakteristischen Kurve wird wesentlich beeinflußt durch die Wahl der therapeutischen Maßnahmen. So ließ sich insbesondere der Prozentsatz potentiell kurativ behandelter Patienten mit hochmalignen Lymphomen durch eine Intensivierung der Chemotherapie in den letzten Jahren deutlich erhöhen.

Voraussetzungen und Prinzipien der Therapie der Non-Hodgkin-Lymphome

Parallel zur Sicherung der Diagnose bildet die umfassende Diagnostik zur Feststellung des initial vorliegenden Stadiums eine Grundvoraussetzung jeglichen therapeutischen Vorgehens. Ziel der entsprechenden Untersuchungen muß es vorrangig sein, eine lokalisierte Erkrankung abzugrenzen von einer auch nur beginnenden Aussaat über den Entstehungsort des Tumors hinaus. So sind neben der klinischen Statuserhebung und der Bestimmung der relevanten Laboratoriumsparameter eine röntgenologische (einschließlich Computertomographie), sonographische und gegebenenfalls szintigraphische Untersuchung von Thorax und Abdomen, eine röntgenologische und/oder endoskopische Untersuchung des Magendarmtraktes sowie eine zyto- und histologische Analyse des Knochenmarks erforderlich. Insbesondere ist ein streng lokalisiertes Stadium I/I_E unbedingt abzusichern durch die konsequente Ausschöpfung der modernen bildgebenden und endoskopischen Verfahren einschließlich der Lymphangioadenographie, durch Liquoruntersuchung und Leberbiopsie sowie gegebenenfalls sogar durch eine explorative («staging»-)Laparotomie, sofern eine Bestrahlung ohne zusätzliche Chemotherapie vorgesehen ist.

Entwicklungen in der Therapie lokoregional begrenzter Erkrankungen

Ausgehend von der Annahme einer unifokalen Entstehung der NHL darf erwartet werden, daß eine diagnostisch gesicherte lokoregional begrenzte Lymphommanifestation durch lokale, insbesondere radiotherapeutische Maßnahmen in anhaltende Vollremission gebracht und damit geheilt werden kann. Diese Auffassung wird belegt durch zahlreiche internationale Erfahrungen, wonach etwa 60–90% der Patienten mit NHL niedrigen Malignitätsgrades im streng lokalisierten Ausbreitungsstadium I/I_E nach Involved- oder Extended-field-Bestrahlung nach 5 Jahren noch in Vollremission sind [27]. Ähnliches gilt auch für einige hochmaligne, nämlich die zentro-(CB) und immunoblastischen (IB) Lymphome, wobei allerdings die Vollremissionsstabilität beim immunoblastischen Lymphom geringer ist als beim zentroblastischen Typ. Nach neueren Untersuchungen darf bei Patienten im Stadium I/I_E mit einer anhaltenden Rezidivfreiheit nach alleiniger Radiotherapie nur dann gerechnet werden, wenn eine «pathologische» Stadiendiagnostik (PS) vorausgegangen ist, die eine Staging-Laparotomie mit Splenektomie, Leberpunktion und -Keilexzision nebst Biopsien multipler intraabdomineller Lymphknoten einschließt. Wird das Stadium I/I_E dagegen nur durch weniger invasive diagnostische Maßnahmen festgelegt («klinische» Stadiendiagnostik, CS), sind bei bis zur Hälfte der Patienten Rezidive binnen 2–5 Jahren zu erwarten [6, 12]. Basierend auf diesen Erfahrungen wird inzwischen an mehreren Zentren bei Patienten im nicht vollständig gesicherten Stadium CS I/I_E eine z. T. durchaus intensive Induktionspolychemotherapie durchgeführt [6, 9, 28], die durch eine adjuvante Radiotherapie ergänzt werden kann. Die mit diesem Vorgehen erreichbaren Vollremissions- (90–95%) und Rezidivfreiheitsquoten (70–100% nach 2–5 Jahren) entsprechen den günstigen Ergebnissen der Radiotherapie bei Patienten im «pathologisch» definierten Stadium PS I/I_E [12]. Vor allem im Stadium II/II_E oder bei Vorliegen einer B-Symptomatik, die anscheinend eine okkulte Überschreitung der Grenzen des lokoregionalen Befalls signalisiert, birgt die alleinige Radiotherapie ein hohes Rezidivrisiko in sich und kann daher nicht mehr uneingeschränkt empfohlen werden. Eine Ausnahme bildet lediglich das besonders strahlensensitive zentroblastisch-zentrozytische (CB-CC) Lymphom, das auch bei einem Teil der Patienten im fortgeschrittenen Stadium III durch umfassende radiotherapeutische Maßnahmen noch dauerhaft unter Kontrolle gebracht werden kann; Voraussetzung dafür scheint jedoch eine insgesamt geringe Tumormasse zu sein. Die starke Neigung lymphoblastischer (LB) Lymphome zur frühen Generalisation mit häufig nachfolgender Entwicklung einer akuten Lymphoblastenleukämie schließt auch im lokoregional streng begrenzten Initialstadium dieser Erkrankung eine alleinige Radiotherapie aus. Ob bzw. inwieweit zumindest bei den streng lokalisierten hochmalignen NHL das kurative Potential einer initialen Radiotherapie durch eine adjuvante Polychemotherapie verstärkt und damit die Heilungschance erhöht werden kann, wird derzeit noch in einer randomisierten Therapiestudie geprüft [32].

Neue Ansätze zur Therapie fortgeschrittener niedrig-maligner Non-Hodgkin-Lymphome

Bis vor wenigen Jahren wurde für die Therapie der fortgeschrittenen niedrig-malignen NHL das expektative Konzept («watch and wait») generell befolgt, das den Einsatz einer wenig intensiven Chemotherapie erst bei Progredienz und dann mit nur palliativer Intention beinhaltete [5, 11, 29]. Dieses Konzept bildete auch die Grundlage der in der näheren prospektiven Beobachtungsstudie der Kieler Lymphomgruppe [4] verfolgten Strategie. In dem Bemühen, die Prognose dieser Erkrankungen zu verbessern und eventuell sogar eine Heilung zu erreichen, sind inzwischen mehrere neue therapeutische Ansätze untersucht worden.

So wurde bei der chronischen lymphatischen Leukämie vom B-Zellentyp (B-CLL) in Abhängigkeit vom Initialstadium der Erkrankung eine Chemotherapie abgestufter Intensität erprobt [15]. Dieser Studie lag die Stadieneinteilung von Binet zugrunde, die bei unbeeinträchtigter Erythro- und Thrombozytopoese je nach Ausdehnung des Lymphknotenbefalls ein Stadium A oder B (Befall von weniger oder mehr als drei Regionen) unterscheidet. Dagegen begründen eine Anämie und/oder Thrombozytopenie definierten Schweregrades das Vorliegen des Stadiums C. Durch den Einsatz von Chlorambucil im Stadium A ließ sich die Prognose gegenüber der unbehandelten Kontrollgruppe nicht relevant verbessern. Auch Patienten im Stadium B, die mit COP (Cyclophosphamid, Vincristin, Prednison) behandelt worden waren, ließen keine höhere Überlebenswahrscheinlichkeit erkennen als diejenigen, die lediglich Chlorambucil erhalten hatten. Im prognostisch ungünstigsten Stadium C war dagegen ein modifiziertes CHOP-Schema (COP + Adriamycin, 25 mg/m^2) dem COP-Schema deutlich überlegen, was durch eine Verbesserung der 2-Jahres-Überlebensquote von 44% in dem COP-behandelten Kollektiv gegenüber 77% in der CHOP-behandelten Gruppe zum Ausdruck kam.

Bereits im Verlauf der Beobachtungsstudie der Kieler Lymphomgruppe (Abb. 1) [4] war die ungünstige Prognose des zentrozytischen (CC) Lymphoms aufgefallen, die mit einer medianen Überlebenszeit von etwa 2 1/2 Jahren wesentlich schlechter war als diejenige des LP-Immunozytoms (LP-IC) (rund 4 Jahre) sowie der B-CLL oder des CB-CC-Lymphoms (jeweils rund 5 Jahre). In einer nachfolgenden prospektiven randomisierten Therapiestudie über das fortgeschrittene CC-Lymphom wurde – bei sofortigem Einsatz einer Polychemotherapie nach Abschluß der initialen Stadiendiagnostik – die Effizienz des COP – mit derjenigen des (durch den Gehalt an Adriamycin) intensiveren CHOP-Schemas verglichen. Allerdings ergab sich weder bezüglich der Vollremissionsquote oder Remissionsdauer noch der Rezidiv- oder Tumortodhäufigkeit ein signifikanter Unterschied zwischen beiden Therapiegruppen. Die fehlende prognostische Überlegenheit des intensiveren CHOP-Regimes veranschaulichen besonders deutlich die entsprechenden Überlebenswahrscheinlichkeitskurven (Abb. 2a, b) [25]. Im Vergleich zu dem an Umfang und Eingangsmerkmalen sehr ähnlichen Patientenkollektiv der Beobachtungsstudie, das überwiegend nach der expektativen Strategie betreut worden war, ließ sich nur eine geringfügige, nicht signifikante Verbesserung der Prognose durch den sofortigen Einsatz der Polychemotherapie mit COP oder CHOP ermitteln, die in einer Verlängerung der medianen Überlebenszeit um etwa 3 Monate zum Ausdruck kam.

In einer etwa zeitgleich begonnenen Studie einer amerikanischen Arbeitsgruppe an einem nach den üblichen Kriterien (s.o.) noch nicht

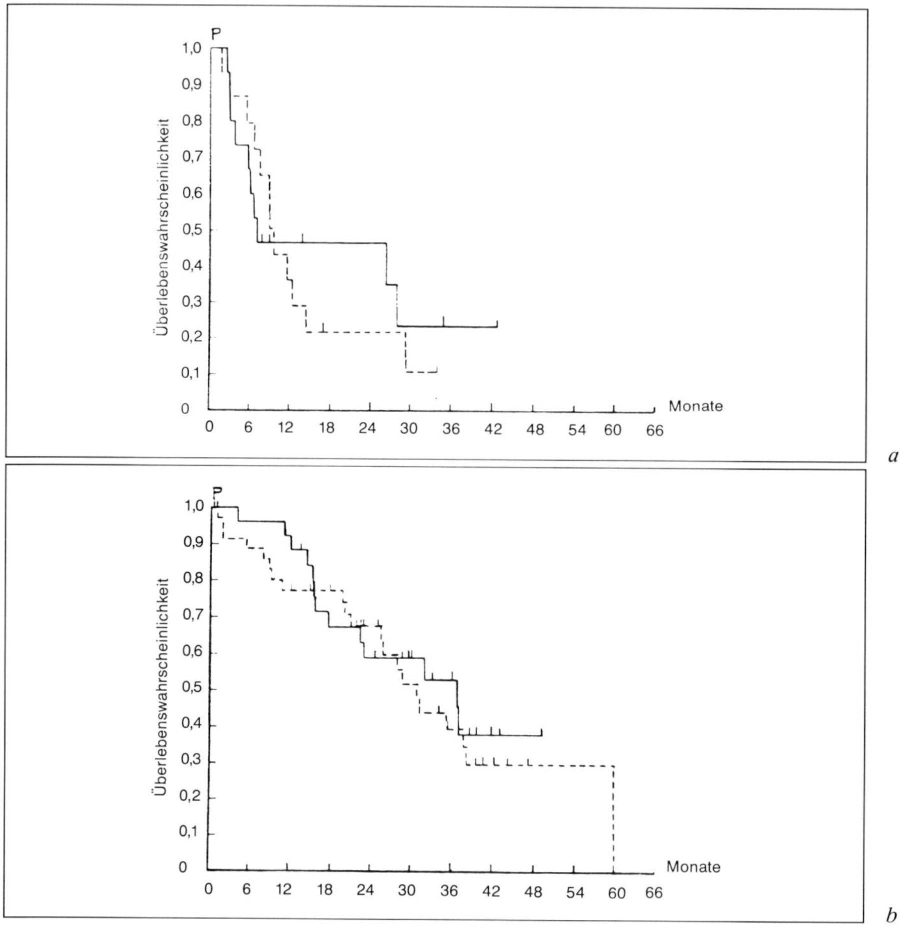

Abb. 2. Überlebenswahrscheinlichkeit der randomisierten Patienten mit zentrozytischem Lymphom in den Stadien III-IV (Ann Arbor-Klassifikation). Ergebnisse der prospektiven Therapiestudie [25]: Vergleich der Induktionstherapie mit dem COP- oder CHOP-Schema. *a.* Gesamtüberlebenswahrscheinlichkeit: — CHOP (n = 26); ..... COP (n = 37). *b.* Rezidivfreiheit: — CHOP (n = 15); ..... COP (n = 15).

behandlungsbedürftigen Patientenkollektiv mit u.a. CB-CC- und CC-Lymphomen sowie LP-IC wurden die Patienten im randomisierten Vergleich entweder nur beobachtet und erst bei Progredienz palliativ behandelt («watch and wait») oder aber bereits initial einer intensiven Induktions-Polychemotherapie (nach dem ProMACE-MOPP-Schema), ergänzt durch eine niedrig dosierte total-lymphatische Bestrahlung, unterworfen [39]. In der Intensivtherapiegruppe wurden bei etwa 78% der Patienten Vollremissionen erreicht, die sich in 86% der Fälle als stabil über etwa 4 Jahre erwiesen, während in der Kontrollgruppe während des Beobachtungszeitraums etwa zwei Drittel der Patienten – meist wiederholt – behandlungsbedürftig wurden. Bei bislang identischer 5-Jahres-Überlebensquote beider Gruppen von 83 bzw. 84% ist ein prognostischer Vorteil der intensiven Induktionstherapie, die bei den Patienten in langjährig anhaltender Vollremission sogar eine mögliche Heilung implizieren könnte, noch nicht erkennbar. Dabei muß allerdings beachtet werden, daß signifikante prognostische Unterschiede bei Patienten mit dieser Gruppe gering proliferierender Tumoren wahrscheinlich erst nach noch längeren Beobachtungszeiten erfaßbar werden.

Die Ergebnisse der skizzierten aktuellen Studien zur Therapie niedrigmaligner NHL bieten sicherlich Ansätze zu einer Verbesserung der Behandlung dieser Erkrankungen, wobei sich zumindest für jüngere Patienten aufgrund ihrer besseren Toleranz gegenüber intensiveren Therapieformen die expektative Strategie bald als überholt erweisen dürfte.

Neue Konzepte zur Therapie der fortgeschrittenen hochmalignen Non-Hodgkin-Lymphome

Im Gegensatz zu den niedrig-malignen NHL ist bei diesen Tumoren der sofortige Einsatz einer intensiven Polychemotherapie unumstritten, da nur eine rasch erreichte stabile Vollremission die Chance der Heilung bietet [5, 8, 11]. Zur Erlangung dieses therapeutischen Zieles stehen mittlerweile zahlreiche Polychemotherapie-Protokolle zur Verfügung (zusammengefaßt in [5, 12], die jedoch einige bedeutsame Unterschiede aufweisen. Die bis Anfang der 80er Jahre eingesetzten Schemata waren gekennzeichnet durch die Applikation einer aus 4 bis 5 Wirkstoffen zusammengesetzten Zytostatika-Kombination, z. B. CHOP, welche dann nach therapiefreiem Intervall, begründet durch die erforderliche Erholung des Knochenmarks, zyklisch wiederholt wurde. Bei den anschließend erprobten und generell als intensiver zu bewertenden Protokollen werden meist sechs oder mehr verschiedene Wirkstoffe (z. B. M-BACOD, COP-BLAM, MACOP-B) kombiniert und in unterschiedlicher Weise gestaffelt verabreicht, so daß sich das therapiefreie Intervall auf weniger als zwei Wochen verkürzt. In einigen weiteren Therapiekonzepten ist darüber hinaus der an den Behandlungserfolg adaptierte sequentielle oder alternierende Einsatz einer zweiten Wirkstoffkombination in der Induktionstherapie vorgegeben wie z. B. bei ProMACE/MOPP [5, 12], Pro-MACE/CytaBOM [5, 12], COP-BLAM/IMVP-16 [16], VAMP/EEE [35]. Eine andere Variante einer Induktionsbehandlung, die derzeit in einer oligozentrischen Studie erprobt wird [21], ist charakterisiert durch die Beschränkung der Chemotherapie auf insgesamt vier Zyklen zweier alternierend verabreichter Schemata (nCHOP/IVEP), gefolgt vom frühzeitigen Einsatz einer Involved-field-Radiotherapie.

Die bisher international gewonnenen Therapieergebnisse (Vollremissionsquoten von ca. 60–85%, rezidivfreies Überleben von 40–70% über mindestens 2 Jahre) lassen zweifelsfrei einen Gewinn an Vollremissionen durch diese modernen, differenzierteren Schemata erkennen. Dagegen ist die Beurteilung der Remissionsstabilität und damit die Einschätzung der Rate endgültiger Heilungen vor allem wegen der sich erheblich unterscheidenden Nachbeobachtungszeiten noch sehr problematisch. Darüber hinaus muß bei der vergleichenden Beurteilung derartiger Daten beachtet werden, inwieweit die Patientenkollektive der einzelnen Studien hinsichtlich ihrer Zusammensetzung (z. B. Homo- oder Heterogenität der Lymphom-Entitäten, Prinzipien ihrer histologischen Zuordnung, Alters- und/oder Stadienverteilung) überhaupt vergleichbar sind und ob die Daten uni- oder multizentrisch gewonnen wurden [2]. Das Beispiel einer prospektiven randomisierten Therapiestudie zur Therapie hochmaligner NHL, die z. Zt. in der Bundesrepublik Deutschland und Österreich durchgeführt wird, zeigt [16], daß bei den nach zentraler histopathologischer Diagnosestellung zwar nach einheitlichen Konzepten, jedoch multizentrisch untersuchten und behandelten Patienten das remissionsinduzierende Potential der CHOP-Therapie dem des COP-BLAM/IMVP-16-Schemas durchaus vergleichbar ist. Wie die Überlebenswahrscheinlichkeitskurven (Abb. 3a, b) erkennen lassen, befindet sich allerdings ein großer Teil der COP-BLAM/IMVP-16-behandelten Patienten noch in der späten Therapie – bzw. frühen Nachbeobachtungsphase. Erst wenn das Niveau eines die Heilungsquote signalisierenden Kurvenplateaus durch die Mehrheit der Patienten definiert ist, könnte eine potentielle prognostische Überlegenheit eines risikoadaptierten Mehrkomponenten-Flexi-Protokolls gegenüber einer zyklischen Standardtherapie erkennbar werden. Dies gilt insbesondere auch für die prognostische Einschätzung der in diesem Studienprotokoll randomisiert eingesetzten adjuvanten Radiotherapie.

Besondere Beachtung muß immer noch den Patienten gelten, welche mit den bisher erprobten therapeutischen Maßnahmen nicht geheilt werden können. Dabei wird die definitive Quote geheilter Patienten nicht nur durch

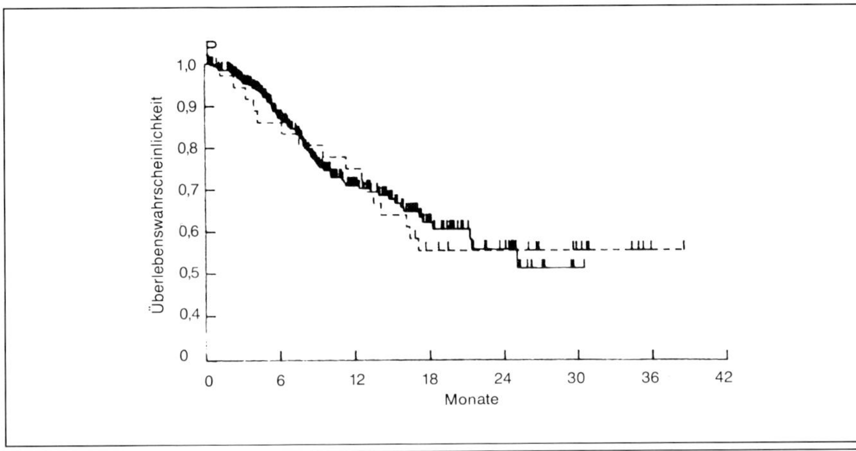

a

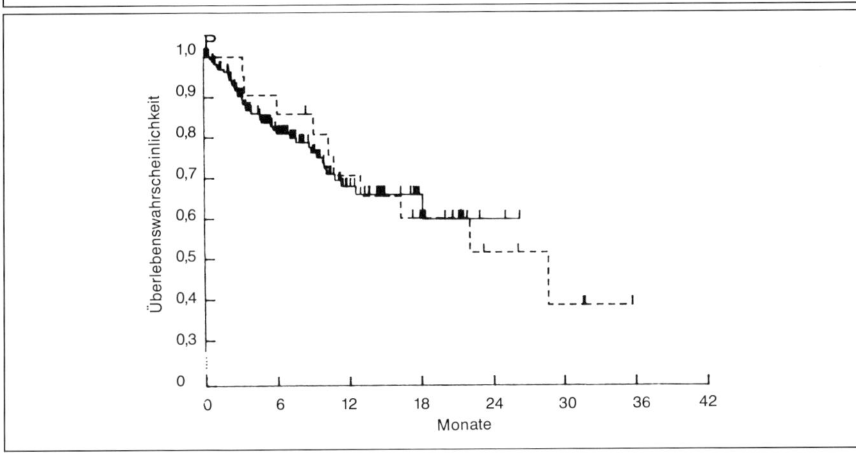

b

Abb. 3. Überlebenswahrscheinlichkeit der Patienten mit hochmalignem NHL Stadien II-IV (Ann Arbor-Klassifikation). Ergebnisse einer Zwischenauswertung der prospektiven Therapiestudie [16]: Induktionstherapie mit dem CHOP- oder COP-BLAM/IMVP-16-Protokoll. *a.* Gesamtüberlebenswahrscheinlichkeit: — COP-BLAM/IMVP-16 (n = 337); ..... CHOP (n = 37). *b.* Rezidivfreiheit: — COP-BLAM/IMVP-16 (n = 168); ..... CHOP (n = 15).

den Anteil (mindestens 30%) der bereits gegenüber der Induktionstherapie refraktären Patienten bestimmt, sondern auch durch die bei etwa 20–30% der Patienten nach Erreichen einer Vollremission auftretenden Rezidive weiter begrenzt. Für beide Gruppen lassen sich trotz intensiver internationaler Bemühungen aus den vielfältigen Ansätzen einer Sekundärbehandlung, z. B. mit vorher noch nicht applizierten Zytostatika [38] sowie sehr intensiven und/oder hochtoxischen Wirkstoffkombinationen [19], noch keine Therapieempfehlungen ableiten, die die insgesamt ungünstige Prognose derartiger Patienten nennenswert und dauerhaft verbessern könnten.

Perspektiven der Therapie der Non-Hodgkin-Lymphome

Aus den bisher bei der Therapie der NHL international gesammelten Erfahrungen ergeben sich einige Perspektiven für zukünftige Therapiekonzepte. So lassen die konventionellen Therapiestrategien noch einen Spielraum zur Verbesserung der Heilungschancen erkennen. In den streng lokalisierten Stadien I/I_E hochmaligner NHL könnten die Ergebnisse der Radiotherapie durch den Einsatz einer adjuvanten Chemotherapie verbessert werden, sofern sich deren prognostische Relevanz belegen läßt. Allerdings legen die erwähnten hervorragenden Ergebnisse einer initialen Polychemotherapie, evtl. ergänzt durch eine adjuvante Radiotherapie, die Möglichkeit nahe, daß sich eine derartige Therapiestrategie bei CR- und IB-Lymphomen im Stadium I/I_E gegenüber der initialen Radiotherapie als überlegen erweist. Bei fortgeschrittenen niedrig-malignen NHL könnte die Identifizierung von therapiesensitiven bzw. von Hochrisiko-Untergruppen dazu beitragen, sehr intensive Therapieformen gezielt einzusetzen. Bei fortgeschrittenen hochmalignen NHL sind u.U. noch Modifikationen der in den letzten Jahren entwickelten und erprobten Chemotherapieschemata vorstellbar. Außerdem werden sowohl die frühzeitig konsolidierende als auch die adjuvante Radiotherapie einen festen Platz in der Behandlungsstrategie einnehmen müssen, wenn sich aus Therapiestudien der Beweis für die prognostische Wertigkeit derartiger Verfahrensweisen ableiten läßt. Auch hier kommt vermutlich der Identifikation von Untergruppen mit hohem Risiko eine besondere Bedeutung zu.

Einige weitere klinische und experimentelle Beboachtungen bieten bereits Ansätze zu einer sinnvollen Modifikation konventioneller Chemotherapiestrategien. So könnte der konsequente Einsatz der biologisch möglichen Wirkstoffhöchstdosen in der jeweiligen Zytostatika-Kombination, d.h. die Beachtung der maximalen «relative dose intensity» [11], die Heilungschance merklich verbessern. Darüber hinaus sind die einzelnen Wirkstoffe einer Kombination für die Remissionsinduktion nicht gleichwertig, und zumindest im Tiermodell ist anscheinend eine höhere Zytostatika-Dosis für die Heilung erforderlich als allein für die Remissionsinduktion. Zusätzlich könnte die Applikationsform insofern bedeutsam sein, als die kontinuierliche Infusion einzelner Wirkstoffe wirksamer zu sein scheint als die Bolusinjektion [3]. Die aus diesen Beboachtungen abgeleitete Zielvorstellung einer Intensivierung der Induktionschemotherapie hat notwendigerweise eine entsprechende Verbesserung der supportiven Therapie zur Voraussetzung, wobei die Verabreichung von Faktoren, die die Hämatopoese, insbesondere die Granulozytopoese stimulieren («colony stimulating factors») CSF [24, 26, 37] an Bedeutung gewinnt. Desgleichen sollte für jüngere Patienten mit erkennbar hohem Rezidivrisiko (z.B. Vorliegen eines niedrig-malignen NHL oder eines nur unvollständig oder verzögert auf die Induktionstherapie ansprechenden hochmalignen NHL) der frühzeitige Einsatz der Chemotherapie mit oder ohne Ganzkörperbestrahlung in supravitaler Dosierung mit nachfolgender autologer Knochenmarktransplantation erwogen werden [18, 36]. Darüber hinaus bleibt zu hoffen, daß derzeit experimentell erprobte Strategien klinisch entsprechend modifiziert und abgesichert werden können und damit Eingang in Standardtherapiekonzepte finden werden. Hierzu zählt neben der Entwicklung neuer Zytostatika vor allem die Integration von Immunmodulatoren [13], z.B. bestimmter Zytokine (Interferon, in Sonderfällen Interleukin-2 [30] oder monoklonaler Antikörper (anti-idiotypische Antikörper [10, 20] oder Toxin-Konjugate [14]. In die Entwicklung zukünftiger Therapiestrategien müssen außerdem eine Reevaluierung der bisher identifizierten und die Definition neuer Risikofaktoren für die einzelnen Entitäten bzw. Lymphomgruppen einbezogen werden. Neben den etablierten, das langfristige Überleben signifikant beeinflussenden Risikofaktoren (z.B. Alter und Allgemeinzustand der Patienten, Ausmaß des Tumorbefalls sowie Präsenz von Allgemeinsymptomen und einer erhöhten Serumaktivität der Laktatdehyrogenase) wird die potentielle prognostische Relevanz einiger Tumormerkmale zu überprüfen sein. Beispielhaft lassen sich hierfür chromosomale Veränderungen [1, 31], der Immunphänotyp [23, 33] und die Proliferationsaktivität sowie die in vitro bestimmte Sensitivität oder Resistenz gegenüber Zytostatika oder Immunmodulatoren nennen.

Die langfristige klinische Relevanz der aufgezeigten Perspektiven zur Entwicklung effizienterer Therapiekonzepte der NHL kann dann aber erst durch prospektive randomisierte Studien ermittelt werden.

Literatur

1 Aisenberg, A.C.; Wilkes, B.M.; Jacobson, J.O.; Harris, N.L.: Immunoglobulin gene rearrangements in adult non-Hodgkin's lymphoma. Am. J. Med. *82:* 738–744 (1987).

2 Armitage, J.O.; Cheson, B.D.: Interpretation of clinical trials in diffuse large-cell lymphoma. J. clin. Oncol. *6:* 1335–1347 (1988).

3 Boyd, D.B.; Coleman, M.; Papish, S.W., et al.: COPBLAM III: Infusional combination chemotherapy for diffuse large-cell lymphoma. J. clin. Oncol. *6:* 425–433 (1988).

4 Brittinger, G.; Bartels, H.; Common, H., et al. for the Kiel Lymphoma Study Group: Clinical and prognostic relevance of the Kiel classification of non-Hodgkin lymphomas results of a prospective multicenter study by the Kiel Lymphoma Study Group. Hematol. Oncol. *2:* 269–306 (1984).

5 Brittinger, G.; Meusers, P.; Engelhard, M.: Strategien der Behandlung von Non-Hodgkin-Lymphomen. Internist *27:* 485–497 (1986).

6 Bron, D.; Stryckmans, P.: Role of chemotherapy for localized non-Hodgkin's lymphoma? Eur. J. Cancer clin. Oncol. *23:* 459–463 (1987).

7 Cabanillas, F.; Velasquez, W.S.; McLaughlin, P., et al.: Results of recent salvage chemotherapy regimens for lymphoma and Hodgkin's disease. Semin. Hematol. *25:* Suppl. 2, S. 47–50 (1988).

8 Coleman, M.; Gerstein, G.; Topilow, A., et al.: Advances in chemotherapy for large cell lymphoma. Semin. Hematol. *24:* Suppl. 1, S. 8–20 (1987).

9 Connors, J.M.; Klimo, P.; Fairey, R.N.; Voss, N.: Brief chemotherapy and involved field radiation therapy for limited-stage, histologically aggressive lymphoma. Ann. Intern. Med. *107:* 25–30 (1987).

10 DePinho, R.A.; Feldman, L.B.; Scharff, M.D.: Tailor-made monoclonal antibodies. Ann. Intern. Med. *104:* 225–233 (1986).

11 De Vita jr., V.T.; Hubbard, S.M.; Longo, D.L.: The chemotherapy of lymphomas: Looking back, moving forward – The Richard and Hinda Rosenthal Foundation Award Lecture. Cancer Res. *47:* 5810–5824 (1987).

12 De Vita jr., V.T.; Hubbard, S.M.; Young, R.C.; Longo, D.L.: The role of chemotherapy in diffuse aggressive lymphomas. Semin. Hematol. *25:* Suppl. 2, S. 2–10 (1988).

13 Fauci, A.S.; Rosenberg, S.A.; Sherwin, S.A., et al.: Immunomodulators in clinical medicine. Ann. Intern. Med. *106:* 421–433 (1987).

14 Fitzgerald, D.J.; Willingham, M.C.; Cardarelli, C.O., et al.: A monoclonal antibody-pseudomonas toxin conjugate that specifically kills multidrug-resistant cells. Proc. Natl. Acad. Sci. *84:* 4288–4292 (1987).

15 French Cooperation Group: Effectiveness of 'CHOP' regimen in advanced untreated chronic lymphocytic leukaemia. Lancet *i:* 1346–1349 (1986).

16 Gerhartz, H.H.; Wilmanns, W.; Brittinger, G. et al.: Risiko-adaptierte Therapie hochmaligner non-Hodgkin Lymphome mit COP-BLAM/IMVP-16: eine prospektive multizentrische Studie. Onkologie *12:* (1989).

17 Hagberg, H.; Cavallin-Ståhl, E.; Lind, J.: Ifosfamide and etoposide as salvage therapy for non-Hodgkin's lymphoma. Scand. J. Haematol. *36:* 61–64 (1985).

18 Hartmann, T.P.O.; Biron, P.; Cahn, J.Y., et al.: High-dose therapy and autologous bone marrow transplantation in partial remission after first-line induction therapy for diffuse non-Hodgkin's lymphoma. J. clin. Oncol. *6:* 1118–1124 (1988).

19 Ho, A.D.; Del Valle, F.; Rückle, R., et al.: Novantrone and high-dose Ara-C (NOAC) as salvage therapy for resistant non-Hodgkin lymphoma. Blut *57:* 252 (1988).

20 Houghton, A.; Scheinberg, D.: Monoclonal antibodies in the treatment of hematopoietic malignancies. Semin. Hematol. *25:* Suppl. 3, S. 23–29 /1988).

21 Köppler, H.; Pflüger, K.H.; Havemann, K., et al.: Treatment of high grade non-Hodgkin lymphoma: Results of a phase II and a phase III trial. Blut *57:* 220 (1988).

22 Lennert, K.; Mohri, N.; Stein, H.; Kaiserling, E.: The histopathology of malignant lymphoma. Br. J. Haematol. *31:* 192–203 (1975).

23 Lippmann, S.M.; Miller, T.P.; Spier, C.M., et al.: The prognostic significance of the immunotype in diffuse large-cell lymphoma: A comparative study of the T-cell and B-cell phenotype. Blood *72:* 436–441 (1988).

24 Metcalf, D.: The granulocyte-macrophage colony stimulating factors. Cell *43:* 5–6 (1985).

25 Meusers, P.; Engelhard, M.; Bartels, H., et al.: Multicenter randomized therapeutic trial for advanced centrocytic lymphoma: Anthracycline does not improve the prognosis. Hematol. Oncol. (im Druck).

26 Morstyn, G.; Souza, L.M.; Keech, J., et al.: Effect of granulocyte colony stimulating factor on neutropenia induced by cytotoxic chemotherapy. Lancet *i:* 667–671 (1988).

27 Paryani, S.B.; Hoppe, R.T.; Cox, R.S., et al.: Analysis of non-Hodgkin's lymphomas with nodular and favorable histologies, stages I and II. Cancer *52:* (1983).

28 Prestidge, B.R.; Horning, S.J.; Hoppe, R.T.: Combined modality therapy for stage I–II large celle lymphoma. J. Rad. Oncol. Biol. Phys. *15:* 633–639 (1988).

29 Rosenberg, S.A.: The low-grade non-Hodgkin's lymphomas: Challenges and opportunities. J. clin. Oncol. *3:* 299–310 (1985).

30 Rosenberg, S.A.; Lotze, M.T.; Muul, L.M., et al.: Observations on the systemic administration of autologous lymphokine-activated killer cells and recombinant interleukin-2 to patient with metastatic cancer. New Engl. J. Med. *313:* 1485–1492 (1985).

31 Rowley, J.D.: Chromosome studies in the non-Hodgkin's lymphomas: The role of the 14; 18 translocation. J. clin. Oncol. *6:* 919–925 (1988).

32 Sack, H.: Therapie der Non-Hodgkin-Lymphome hoher Malignität des Stadiums I, der niedrig-malignen Non-Hodgkin-Lymphome der Stadien I und II und der centrocytischen-centroblastischen Lymphome der Stadien I–III. Studienprotokoll (1985).

33 Schuurman, H.-J.; Huppes, W.; Verdonck, L.F., et al.: Immunophenotyping of non-Hodgkin's lymphoma. Correlation with relapse-free survival. Am. J. Pathol. *131:* 102–111 (1988).

34 Stansfeld, A.G.; Diebold, J.; Kapanci, Y., et al.: Updated Kiel classification for lymphomas. Lancet *i:* 292–293 (1988).

35 Stuart, N.S.A.; Blackledge, G.R.P.; Child, J.A., et al.: A new approach to the treatment of advanced high-grade non-Hodgkin's lymphoma – intensive two-phase chemotherapy. Cancer Chemother. Pharmacol. *22:* 141–146 (1988).

36 Takvorian, T.; Canellos, G.P.; Ritz, J., et al.: Prolonged disease-free survival after autologous bone marrow transplantation in patients with non-Hodgkin's lymphoma with a poor prognosis. New Engl. J. Med. *316:* 1499–1505 (1987).

37 Vadhan-Raj, S.; Buescher, S.; LeMaistre, A., et al.: Stimulation of hematopoiesis in patients with bone marrow failure and in patients with malignancy by recombinant human granulocyte-macrophage colony-stimulating factor. Blood *72:* 134–141 (1988).

38 Warrell, P.; Danieu, L.; Coonley, C.J.; Atkins, C.: Salvage chemotherapy of advanced lymphoma with investigational drugs: Mitoguazone, gallium nitrate, and etoposide. Cancer Treat. Rep. *71:* 47–51 (1987).

39 Young, R.C.; Longo, D.L.; Glatstein, E., et al.: The treatment of indolent lymphomas: Watchful waiting V aggressive combined modality treatment. Semin. Hematol. *25:* Suppl. 2, S. 11–16 (1988).

Dr. med. M. Engelhard, Medizinische Universitätsklinik,
Hufelandstraße 55, D-4300 Essen (BRD)

Beitr Onkol, vol. 36, pp. 58–65 (Karger, Basel 1989)

Therapie der hochmalignen Non-Hodgkin-Lymphome bei älteren Patienten

R. Kuse[a], A. Calavrezos[a], Ruth Sonnen[a], H.-P. Heilmann[b]

[a] Hämatologische Abteilung,
[b] Institut für Strahlentherapie des Allgemeinen Krankenhauses St. Georg, Hamburg

Einleitung

Obwohl hochmaligne Non-Hodgkin-Lymphome sehr häufig im höheren Lebensalter vorkommen, sind Patienten jenseits des 60. Lebensjahres in Therapiestudien zu höchstens 25% vertreten. In den letzten Jahren mehren sich aber Publikationen, die sich vorrangig mit den Behandlungsergebnissen bei älteren Patienten befassen, wobei die Trenngrenze zu den jüngeren Jahrgängen mit 60, 65, 70 und 80 Jahren angegeben werden. Die mediane Überlebenszeit liegt in allen Gruppen unter 36 Monaten [1, 3, 6, 10, 13, 15, 21, 22].

Als besonders problematisch erweist es sich hierbei, daß eine reduzierte Zytostatika-Toleranz im höheren Lebensalter infolge veränderter Bioverfügbarkeit und Pharmakokinetik sowie einer verzögerten hämatopoetischen Regeneration [2, 14] einer angestrebten, möglichst intensiven Therapie entgegen steht.

Unsere Arbeitsgruppe hat daher schon frühzeitig versucht, durch die sequentielle Kombination von dosisreduzierter Polychemo- und Großfeldradiotherapie die Toxizität zu senken und dennoch schnelle und stabile Remissionen zu induzieren [17, 18].

Patienten und Methoden

Datenkörper

Es wurden 246 Patienten aus dem Zeitraum 1976–1987 untersucht und behandelt (Tab. 1). Die Trenngrenze zum höheren Lebensalter wurde bei 60 Jahren gezogen, da die EDV-gestützte Analyse der Altersdekaden einen signifikanten prognostischen Unterschied für

Patienten diesseits und jenseits des 60. Lebensjahres ergeben hatte. Zwischen der 7. und 8. Altersdekade bestand kein Unterschied (Abb. 1). Die vom Lymphknotenregister in Kiel primär oder konsilidarisch diagnostizierten histologischen Subtypen wurden zusammengefaßt ausgewertet, da sie prognostisch ähnlich waren. Lymphoblastische und periphere T-Zell-Lymphome wurden nicht einbezogen. In den Stadien I und II zeigten 57% der Patienten einen primär extranodalen Befall. In 32% der Fälle, vorwiegend in den Stadien III und IV, lag eine große Tumormasse vor. Über 60% der älteren Patienten waren polymorbide.

Tabelle 1. Patienten-Daten

	gesamt	≦60 Jahre		>60 Jahre	
		n	%	n	%
Alle Patienten	246	115	47	131	53
Stadium I	94	50	43	44	34
Stadium II	77	31	27	46	35
Stadien III + IV	75	34	30	41	31
Immunoblastisch	81	–	–	–	–
Centroblastisch	109	–	–	–	–
Unklassifizierbar	56	–	–	–	–
Altersmedian aller Patienten	62 J.	46 (16–60)		71 (61–88)	
Stadien I + II		42		70	
Stadien III + IV		48		71	

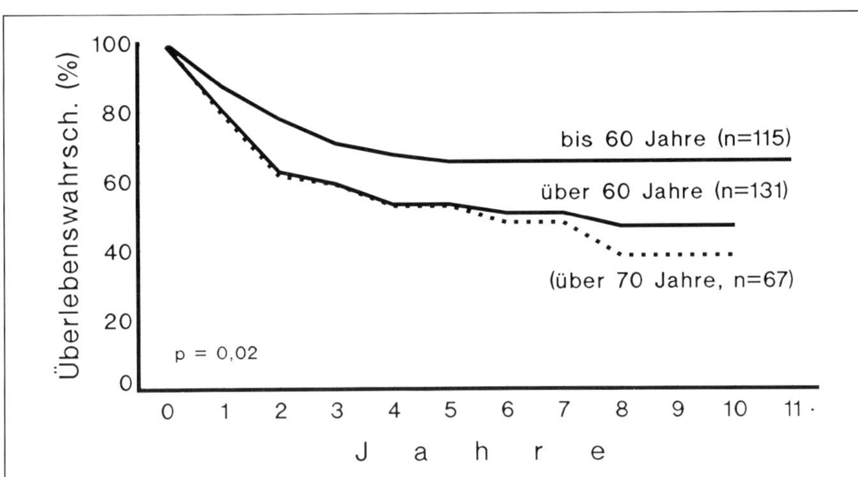

Abb. 1. Überlebenswahrscheinlichkeit für Patienten bis zum 60. Lebensjahr und jenseits des 60. Lebensjahres.

Behandlung

Vor 1976 und in den ersten Jahren danach wurden die Stadien I und II in der Regel radiotherapiert. Häufige Rezidive und Unsicherheiten bei der Stadieneinteilung, insbesondere infolge der begrenzten diagnostischen Belastbarkeit vieler älterer Patienten, führten dazu, daß seit 1979 zunehmend häufiger auch in den Stadien I und II primär die Chemotherapie eingesetzt wurde (Tab. 2) und zwar das CHOP-Schema in 76% aller Fälle. Die Zytostatika wurden in der Regel altersadaptiert auf 70–80% der errechneten Solldosen reduziert. Hierdurch konnte die Knochenmarkstoxizität verringert und die Behandlung in zwei- bis dreiwöchigen Intervallen konsequent und ohne Zeitverluste durchgeführt werden. Nach Erreichen einer Vollremission wurde meist eine konsolidierende Großfeldradiotherapie angeschlossen. Sie erfolgte mit einem 8-MeV-Linearbeschleuniger im oberen Körperabschnitt als «Manteltechnik» mit 30 Gy und im unteren Abschnitt als Abdomenganzbestrahlung mit 25,5 Gy. In Einzelfällen wurde eine zusätzliche lokale «boost»-Dosis von 10 Gy oder eine «involved field»-Therapie mit 30–40 Gy gegeben.

Statistik

Die Überlebenswahrscheinlichkeit wurde nach Kaplan und Meier [16] und nach Cox [9] und Breslow [4] verglichen. Innerhalb klinischer Variablen wurden prognostisch bedeutsame Abstufungen nach Cox und nach dem sogenannten relativen Sterberisiko nach Pike [19] bestimmt und an andere Variablen adjustiert. Waren Patienten infolge Komorbidität verstorben, wurden sie bei der Berechnung der Überlebenswahrscheinlichkeit wie verschollene Fälle gewertet.

Ergebnisse

Die Überlebenswahrscheinlichkeit nach 11 Jahren lag für die Gesamtgruppe bei 56%. Sie wurde für Patienten bis zum 60. Lebensjahr mit 66% und für ältere Patienten mit 47% berechnet. Das mittlere Überleben beträgt

Tabelle 2. Therapiekonzept

Chemotherapie	→ Vollremission:	Radiotherapie konsolidierend
	→ Teilremission:	Radiotherapie kurativ oder Chemotherapie – Intensivierung und Radiotherapie
	→ Nichtremission:	Chemotherapie oder Radiotherapie, teilweise als Palliation
Radiotherapie		nur bei Kontra-Indikation gegen Chemotherapie
Chemo- oder Radiotherapie		als konsolidierende Maßnahme nach totaler Tumorentfernung im sicheren Stadium I, z. B. bei Magen-NHL

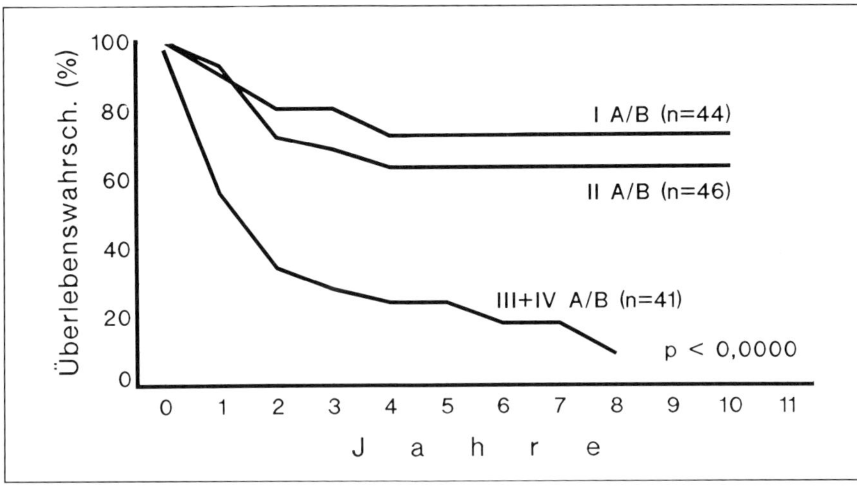

Abb. 2. Überlebenswahrscheinlichkeit und rezidivfreies Überleben.

für die älteren Patienten 84 Monate. Ein Plateau besteht für die jüngeren Patienten vom 5., für die älteren Patienten vom 8. Jahr an (Abb. 1). Das rezidivfreie Überleben für die Gesamtgruppe beträgt 47%, wobei noch nach 9 Jahren ein Rezidiv registriert wurde (Abb. 2). Die risikoadaptierte Behandlung führte in den Stadien I und II durch Radiotherapie in 40%, durch Chemotherapie in 78% und durch die sequentielle Kombination von Chemo- und Radiotherapie in 76% zu ununterbrochenen Remissionen (Abb. 3). Eine Chemotherapie allein hatten meistens Patienten im Stadium I erhalten, deren Tumor zum Beispiel durch Magenteilresektion völlig entfernt worden war. Für das Stadium I ergab sich nach zehn Jahren eine Überlebenswahrscheinlichkeit von 74% und für das Stadium II von 63%, während diese für die Stadien III und IV nach 8 Jahren nur 10% betrug (Abb. 4). Für die jüngeren Altersgruppen wurden 87%, 54% und 48% berechnet.

Diskussion

Die Ergebnisse zeigen, daß ältere Patienten jenseits des 60. Lebensjahres keine wesentlich schlechtere Prognose als jüngere Altersgruppen aufweisen (Abb. 1). Insbesondere in den Stadien I und II ergeben sich ähnliche

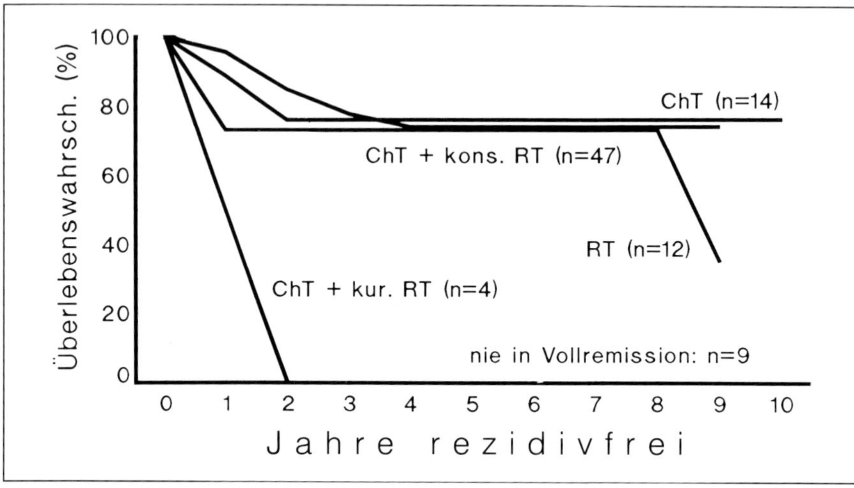

Abb. 3. Rezidivfreies Überleben. ChT = Chemotherapie; ChT + kons. RT = Chemotherapie und konsolidierende Radiotherapie; ChT + kur. RT = Chemotherapie und Radiotherapie mit kurativer Zielsetzung.

Überlebensraten, so daß die Differenz im wesentlichen auf das schlechtere Abschneiden in den mit größerer Tumormasse einhergehenden Stadien III und IV zurückzuführen ist (Abb. 4). Als wesentlicher Faktor für die gegenüber den Angaben in der Literatur verbesserten Überlebensraten unserer älteren Patienten [1, 3, 6, 10, 13, 15, 21, 22] dürfte die sequentielle Kombination von Polychemo- und Großfeldradiotherapie anzusehen sein.

Mit der initialen Chemotherapie auch in den lokalisierten Stadien I und II konnten die Unsicherheiten einer eventuellen unzureichenden Stadieneinteilung, die wegen der eingeschränkten diagnostischen Belastbarkeit älterer Patienten häufig in Kauf genommen werden müssen, ausgeglichen und somit die Risiken einer Unterbehandlung reduziert werden. Die konsolidierende Radiotherapie kann als remissionsstabilisierende Maßnahme im Sinne der Goldie-Coldman-Hypothese [12] zur Minderung der bekanntermaßen hohen Rezidivrate nach CHOP beitragen [5]. Die Notwendigkeit, schnelle und stabile Remissionen zu induzieren, läßt sich auch daran erkennen, daß nur wenige Rezidive wieder in eine zweite anhaltende Remission gebracht werden konnten, wie aus dem geringen Abstand zwischen rezidivfreiem Überleben und Gesamtüberlebensrate hervorgeht (Abb. 2). Es ist bis heute umstritten, ob bei älteren Patienten volle oder reduzierte Zytostatika-Dosen gegeben werden sollen [23]. In unserem Therapiekonzept hat sich die Gabe

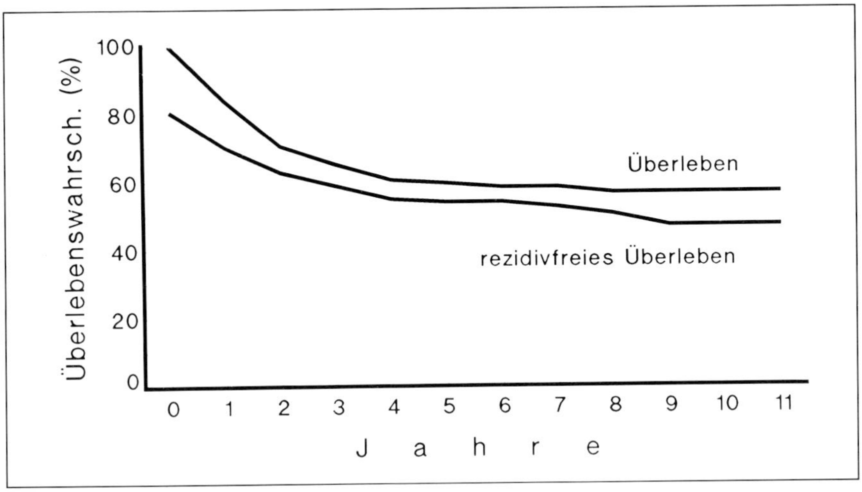

Abb. 4. Überlebenswahrscheinlichkeit in Abhängigkeit von den Stadien.

auf 70–80% reduzierter Solldosen insofern bewährt, als nicht nur die altersbedingt veränderte Bioverfügbarkeit und Pharmakokinetik sowie die verzögerte hämatopoetische Regeneration berücksichtigt werden [2, 14], sondern auch eine konsequente Applikation in kurzen Intervallen ohne Zeitverzögerung möglich ist. Von vorübergehenden Zytopenien unter der Radiotherapie abgesehen, wurden keine wesentlichen Komplikationen beobachtet. Lediglich eine betagte Patientin verstarb an einer Colitis infolge Granulozytopenie nach dem ersten dosisreduzierten CHOP-Zyklus.

Die ungünstigen Ergebnisse für die Stadien III und IV lassen erkennen, daß hier die Grenzen der therapeutischen Belastbarkeit älterer Patienten aufgezeigt werden und für diese meist mit größerer Tumormasse einhergehenden Krankheitsbilder intensivere Behandlungsmaßnahmen erforderlich wären, wie sie in den letzten Jahren bei jüngeren Patienten mit aggressiveren Zytostatik-Kombinationen versucht wurden [3, 8, 11, 20].

Literatur

1 Armitage, J.O.; Potter, J.F.: Aggressive chemotherapy for diffuse histiocytic lymphoma in the elderly: Increased complications with advancing age. J. Am. Geriatr. Soc. *32:* 269–273 (1984).

2 Begg, C.B.; Carbone, P.P.: Clinical trials and drug toxicity in the elderly. The experience of the Eastern Cooperative Oncology Group. Cancer *52:* 1982–1986 (1983).

3 Boyd, D.B.; Coleman, M.; Papish, S.W.; Topilow, A.; Kopel, S.K.; Bernhardt, B.; Files, I.C.; Schwartz, S.; Gaynott, M.; McDermott, D.; Reisman, A.M.; Coleman, B.L.; COP-BLAM III: Infusional combination chemotherapy for diffuse large-cell lymphoma. J. clin. Oncol. *6:* 425–433 (1988).

4 Breslow, N.: A generalized Kruskal-Wallis test for comparing K samples subject to unequal patterns of censorship. Biometrika *57:* 579–595 (1970).

5 Brittinger, G.; Meusers, P.; Engelhard, M.: Strategien der Behandlung von Non-Hodgkin-Lymphomen. Internist *27:* 485–497 (1986).

6 Carbone, A.; Tirelli, U.; Volpe, R.; Zagonel, V.; Manconi R.; Menin, A.; Trovo M.; Grigoletto, E.: Non-Hogdkin's lymphoma in the elderly. A retrospective clinicopathologic study of 50 patients Cancer *57:* 2185–2189 (1986).

7 Coleman, M.; Armitage, J.O.; Gaynor, M.; McDermott, D.; Weissenburger, D.D.; Adler, K.; Beshevkin, M.; Silver, R.T.; Reisman, A.M.; Pasmantier, M.W.: The COP-BLAM programs: Evolving chemotherapy concepts in large cell lymphoma. Semin. Hematol. *25:* Suppl. 2, S. 23–33 (1988).

8 Connors, J.M.; Klimo, R.: MACOP-B chemotherapy for malignant lymphomas and related conditions: 1987 update and additional observations. Semin. Hematol. *25:* Suppl. 2, S. 41–46 (1988).

9 Cox, D.R.: Regression models and life tables (with discussion). J. roy. Statist. Soc. (B) *34:* 187–220 (1972).

10 Dixon, D.O.; Neilan, B.; Jones, S.E.; Lipschitz, D.A.; Miller, Th.P.; Grozea, P.N.; Wilson, H.E.: Effect of age on therapeutic outcome in advanced diffuse histiocytic lymphoma: The Southwest Oncology Group experience. J. clin. Oncol. *4:* 295–305 (1986).

11 Fisher, R.I.; DeVita, V.T.; Hubbard, S.M.; Longo, D.L.; Wesley, R.; Chabner, B.R.; Young, R.C.; Diffuse aggressive lymphomas. Increased survival after alternating flexible sequences of ProMACE and MOPP chemotherapy. Ann. intern. Med. *98:* 304–309 (1983).

12 Goldie, J.H.; Coldman, A.J.; Gudauskas, G.A.: Rationale for the use of alternating non-cross-resistant chemotherapy. Cancer Treat. Rep. *66:* 439–449 (1982).

13 Heinz, R.; Pawlicki, M.; Losonczy, H.; Varbiro, M.; Benedek, S.; Konopka, L.; Krc, I.; Brugiatelli, M.: Initial chemotherapy with an age-adjusted CHOP-schedule in non-Hodgkin lymphomas with unfavorable prognosis. A study of the I.G.C.I. Haematol. *71:* 473–479 (1986).

14 Hirota, Y.; Okamura, S.; Kimura, N.; Shibuay, T.; Niho, Y.: Haematopoiesis in the aged as studied by in vitro colony assay. Eur. J. Haematol. *40:* 83–90 (1988).

15 Hoerni, B.; Sotto, J.J.; Eghbali, H.; Sotto, M.F.; Hoerni-Simon, G.; Pegourié, B.: Non-Hodgkin's malignant lymphomas in patients older than 80. Cancer *61:* 2057–2059 (1988).

16 Kaplan, E.L.; Meier, P.: Nonparametric estimations form incomplete observations. J. Am. stat. Ass. *53:* 457–481 (1958).

17 Kuse, R.; Heilmann, H.-P.; Calavrezos, A.; Hausmann, K.: Sequentielle Polychemotherapie und Großfeld-Radiotherapie von Non-Hodgkin-Lymphomen. Strahlentherapie *161:* 231–238 (1985).

18 Kuse, R.; Calavrezos, A.; Stellbrink, H.J.; Heilmann, H.P.: Langzeitergebnisse bei 172 hochmalignen Nicht-Hodgkin-Lymphomen unter besonderer Berücksichtigung älterer Patienten. Dt. med. Wschr. *112:* 335–340 (1987).

19 Pike, M.C.: Contribution to the discussion on the paper by R. Peto and J. Peto, asymptotically efficient rank invariant test procedures. J. roy. Statist. Soc. (A) *135:* 201–203 (1972).

20 Shipp, M.A.; Harrington, D.P.; Klatt, M.M.; Jochelson, M.S.; Pinkus, G.S.; Marshall, J.L.; Rosenthal, D.S.; Skarin, A.T.; Canellos, G.P.: Identification of major prognostic subgroups of patients with large-cell lymphoma treated with m-BACOD or M-BACOD. Ann. intern. Med. *104:* 757–765 (1986).

21 Solal-Celigny, Ph.; Chastang, C.; Herrera, A.; Desaint, B.; Renoux, M.; Gaulard, Ph.; Bernard, J.F.; Brousse, N.; Boivin, P.: Age as the main prognostic factor in adult aggressive Non-Hodgkin's lymphoma. Am. J. Med. *83:* 1075–1079 (1987).

22 Tirelli, U.; Carbone, A.; Zagonel, V.; Veronesi, A.; Canetta, R.: Non-Hodgkin's lymphomas in the elderly: Prospective studies specifically devised chemotherapy regimens in 66 patients. Europ. J. Cancer clin. Oncol. *23:* 535–540 (1987).

23 Wilmanns, W., Binsack, T.; Sauer, J.: Zytostatische Chemotherapie im höheren Lebensalter. Dt. med. Wschr. *110:* 1959–1962 (1985).

Priv. Doz. Dr. med. Rolf Kuse, Hämatologische Abteilung des Allgemeinen Krankenhauses St. Georg, Lohmühlenstraße 5, D-2000 Hamburg 1 (BRD)

Beitr Onkol, vol. 36, pp. 66–71 (Karger, Basel 1989)

Optimal Timing of Autologous Bone Marrow Transplantation for Patients with Hodgkin's Lymphoma[1]

Angelo M. Carella[a], Angela M. Congiu[a], Patrizio Mazza[b], Giovanna Meloni[c], Lina Mangoni[d], Alessandro Levis[e], Adolfo Porcellini[f], Emilio P. Alessandrino[g], Renato Bassan[h], Paolo Coser[i], Franco Benedetti[k], Sante Tura[b], Franco Mandelli[c], Vittorio Rizzoli[d], Luigi Resegotti[e], Carlo Bernasconi[g], Tiziano Barbui[h], Alberto M. Marmont[a], Eugenio E. Damasio[a]

[a] Division of Hematology, BMT Unit, Genova; [b] Institute of Hematology, Bologna; [c] Institute of Hematology, Roma; [d] Institute of Hematology, Parma; [e] Division of Hematology, Torino; [f] Division of Hematology, Pesaro; [g] Division of Hematology, Pavia; [h] Division of Hematology, Bergamo; [i] Division of Hematology, Bolzano; [j] Institute of Clinical Oncology, Verona, Italy

Introduction

In the last twenty years, the prognosis of patients with advanced Hodgkin's lymphoma has been modified dramatically due to the development of new combination chemotherapy protocols [1, 2].

Although such protocols revolutionized the treatment of advanced Hodgkin's lymphoma, at least one third of the patients do not achieve complete remission or relapse precociously within 12 months. For these patients, the prognosis is very poor, especially for patients resistant to MOPP/ABVD. The more recent conventional salvage therapies do not seem to modify the prognosis of these patients. Because of the poor results with conventional salvage therapies, clinical trials were begun to evaluate the role of high-dose therapy followed by autologous bone marrow transplantation (ABMT) for patients refractory d'emblee to the first line therapy or relapsed to first, second and third-line protocols.

Here we describe our results with 72 patients who received ABMT.

[1] Supported by Associazione Italiana Ricerca sul Cancro (A.I.R.C.), 1989.

Materials and Methods

Patients with advanced Hodgkin's lymphoma received high-dose therapy/ABMT from July 1981 to July 1987; no data collected after July 1987 is included in this analysis. The patients were evaluated at the division of hematology (Genova).

Eligibility criteria included normal bone marrow function in the absence of marrow involvement, Karnofsky performance status 40% and resistance to MOPP and then later to radiation and ABVD or CEP (Lomustine, Etoposide, Prednimustine) [3] or to the alternating regimen of MOPP/ABVD, CEP and radiation, as indicated by either progressive disease during therapy or relapse disease after an initial complete remission.

The clinical characteristics of the patients are shown in table 1. There were 50 males and 22 females with a median age of 26 years (range 12–51). Nodular sclerosis histology was the most prevalent subtype (49 patients). Fifty patients had extranodal disease, and the majority of patients had B symptoms (47 patients). Eleven patients received ABMT in first relapse, 23 had progressive disease while receiving either alternating MOPP/ABVD plus radiation protocol or MOPP followed by ABVD and CEP protocols, and 36 patients had recurrent disease ranging from three months to 45 months after complete remission. Nine out of 36 patients had a first complete remission duration less than one year.

Evaluation and Statistical Analysis

The patients who did never achieve a complete remission after first line treatment and even after second and/or third line therapies, were considered progressive disease patients at transplantation. Relapsing patients were first treated according to a conventional salvage protocol and were classified according to their responsiveness to this protocol as having had either 'resistant relapse' when no response or disease progression were observed immediately before high-dose therapy and autologous transplantation or 'sensitive relapse' when at least a partial response was observed immediately before transplantation [4].

Complete remission was definied as the disappearance of clinical and radiological evidence of Hodgkin's lymphoma. Partial remission was defined as a reduction of 50 percent or more in measurable disease for at least on month.

No complete remission patient received maintenance treatment while patients achieving partial remission always received subsequent radiotherapy.

Disease-free survival was calculated from the day of marrow transplantation (day 0) and was analysed as of February 10, 1988. Actuarial disease-free survival curve was plotted according to the method of Kaplan and Meyer [5].

Supportive Care and Treatment Protocol

In all patients, a central venous catheter was inserted 12 h before high dose therapy. The patients were maintained in single rooms, received prophylactic allopurinol, antiemetics, and oral non adsorbable antibiotics and antimycotics and were given intravenous hydratation until

Table 1. Patient Characteristics

		No. of patients
Total		72
Stage of disease at first presentation	nodes >2	48
	extranodal 1	18
	disease > 1	6
B symptoms		47
Histology	NS	49
	others	23
Karnofsky performance status	70% – 100%	20
	40% – 60%	52
Sites of recurrant Hodgkin's disease	nodes >2	20
	extranodal 1	39
	disease >1	11
Prior therapy	MOPP/ABVD* + RT±CEP	31
	others**	41
Status at the time of HDC/ABMT	first relapse	11
	progressive disease	23
	resistant relapse	13
	sensitive relapse	23
	first complete remission	2

* alternating: MOPP regimen was alternated with ABVD regimen every other month.
** MOPP + RT/ABVD + RT; CcVPP + RT + ABVD±CEP; MA/MA + RT + CEP(CAD).
LP: Lymphocytic predominance; NS: Nodular sclerosis; MC: Mixed cellularity;
LD: Lymphocytic depletion; mED: Mediastinal bulky; CCVPP: Lomustine, Vinblastine, Procarbazine, Prednisone; RT: Radiotherapy; CEP: Lomustine, Etoposide, Prednimustine.
For resistant relapse and sensitive relapse see evaluation and statistical analysis.

day 5 after transplantation. Urine output was maintained at 150 ml/h. The high dose therapies consisted of a modified CVB protocol [6] (table 2).

Results

Tumor Response and Survival

The outcome of high-dose in relation to the patient's characteristics before transplantation is summarized in table 3. Thirty-one (46.2%) patients achieved complete remission with a median duration of 26 months

Table 2. Drug schedules and doses for the chemotherapy regimens used in Italy

Drug regimens	Total dose (mg/mq)		Route	Time
CVB-1				
Cy	6,000	in	i.v.	30 min
VP-16	600	two	i.v.	120 min
BCNU	600	days	i.v.	push (H/D)
				30 min
CVB-2 [10]				
Cy	6,000	in	i.v.	30 min
VP-16	1,000	four	i.v.	120 min
BCNU	800	days	i.v.	push (H/D)
				30 min

Table 3. Results with CVB regimens in patients with advanced Hodgkin's disease

	Evaluable patients	CR	PR	CR+PR	Median CR duration (months)	CCR
First relapse	9	6 (67%)	2	8 (88%)	16	4
Progressive disease	22	10 (46%)	6	16 (72%)	19	7
Resistant relapse	12	3 (25%)	8	11 (92%)	34	2
Sensitive relapse	22	12 (55%)	7	19 (86%)	8	4
First complete remission	2				3	2
	67	31 (46.2%)		54 (80.5%)		19 (61.2%)

and 23 (34.3%) patients achieved a partial remission with a median duration of nine months, for an overall response rate of 80%. Nineteen out of 31 complete responders patients subsequently relapsed after 3 to 28 months (median 7 months). Eleven patients failed to respond and died in progressive disease after 1 to 10 months (median 6 months) after transplantation. The analysis of the progression sites showed that 82% of relapses occurred primarily at the initial site of disease, whereas only 18% occurred in other sites. In no patient relapse occurred in the marrow.

Toxicity

High dose therapy produced significant neutropenia and thrombocytopenia in these heavily pretreated patients. All patients had a white blood cell count less than 0.5 x 10^9/L for a median of 14 days (range 8–34 days) and a platelet count less than 20 x 10^9/L for a median of 20 days (range 14–57). Fever during neutropenia, which warranted intravenous antibiotic and antimycotic therapy, was present in all patient.

There were ten treatment-related deaths; two patients died of Pseudomonas aerguginosa septicemia, and another patient died of Candida pneumonitis; one patient died in complete remission of cerebral hemorrhage two months after transplantation. The autopsy, effected in this case, confirmed the complete remission state. Four patients died of cardiac toxicity and three patients of interstitial pneumonitis. All these cases received ABMT as fourth line therapy.

Eight patients had severe mucositis and three cases had herpes virus simplex generalized infection, well controlled with intravenous Acyclovir.

Nausea, vomiting, liver enzymes and/or alkaline phosphatase elevations were observed in all patients.

Discussion

Hodgkin's lymphoma is a responsive neoplasia both to radiotherapy and chemotherapy. Today, 50–70% of patients with advanced disease can be cured with MOPP or MOPP/ABVD protocols. However, not all patients can be cured with the presently available primary therapies. On the other hand, the optimal management of Hodgkin's lymphoma resistant or relapsing after primary intensive therapy remains to be established. At present, several salvage protocols have been tested for these patients, but the results are controversial and must be interpreted with caution [7].

High-dose therapy and autologous bone marrow transplantation is a promising new approach for these patients. According to the results of pilot studies from the U.S.A. and the European Bone Marrow Transplantation Group (EBMTG), approximately two-third of the end-stage patients can expect to achieve a complete remission after high-dose therapy.

The aim of our study, which was started more than seven years ago, was to improve therapy salvage results in advanced heavily pre-treated patients. In this cooperatice pilot study we showed that it was possible to achieve a high response rate (80%) with a acceptable proportion of early deaths in 72 resistant Hodgkin's lymphoma patients with very bad prognosis. Superimposable results have been obtained by others in similar patients [8, 9].

All these results, as well as those concerning smaller groups of patients, are similar to ours and prove the validity of such procedures in inducing complete remission; however, the high rate of relapse suggests that it may be useful to treat these patients earlier, in first relapse or in second complete remission after standard therapy before ABMT, or in first complete remission in very high risk patients [10].

Clearly, the question of whether high-dose therapy and autologous bone marrow transplantation will eventually supersede new conventional dose salvage chemotherapy, would be answer able only by a controlled clinical trial recently in progress.

References

1 Longo, D.L.; Young, R.C.; Wesley, M., et al.: Twenty years of MOPP therapy for Hodgkin's Disease. J. clin. Oncol. *4:* 1295 (1986).

2 Bonadonna, G.; Valagussa, P.; Santoro, A.: Alternating non-cross-resistant combination chemotherapy or MOPP in stage IV Hodgkin's disease. Ann. Intern. Med. *104:* 739 (1986).

3 Bonadonna, G.; Viviani, S.; Valagussa, P., et al.: Third-line salvage chemotherapy in Hodgkin's disease. Semin. Oncol. *12:* Suppl. 2, p. 23 (1985).

4 Philip, T.; Armitage, J.O.; Spitzer, G., et al.: High-dose therapy and autologous bone marrow transplantation after failure of conventional chemotherapy in adults with intermediate-grade or high-grade non-Hodgkin's lymphoma. New Engl. J. Med. *316:* 1493 (1987).

5 Kaplan, E.L.; Meyer, P.: Nonparametric estimation from incomplete observations. J. Am. Stat. Assoc. *53:* 457 (1958).

6 Jagannath, S.; Dicke, K.A.; Armitage, J.O.; Ann Intern. Med. *104:* 163 (1986).

7 Hagemeister, F.B.; in Fuller, Hagemeister, Sullivan, Velasquez, Hodgkin's disease and Non-Hodgkin's lymphomas in adults and children. p. 285 (New York, Raven Press, 1988).

8 Jagannath, S.; Armitage, J.O.; Velasquez, W.S.; Hagemeister, F.B.; in Fuller, Hagemeister, Sullivan, Velasquez, Hodgkin's disease and Non-Hodgkin's lymphomas in adults and children. p. 440 (New York, Raven Press, 1988).

9 Canellos, G.P.: Bone marrow transplantation as salvage therapy in advanced Hodgkin's disease: Allogeneic or autologous. J. clin. Oncol. *3:* 1451 (1985).

10 Carella, A.M.; Congin, A.; Mazza, P.: J. clin. Oncol. *6:* 1411 (1988).

Dr. A.M. Carella, Division of Hematology, BMT Unit, Ospedale S. Martino, Genova (Italy)

Beitr Onkol, vol. 36, pp. 72–79 (Karger, Basel 1989)

Hochdosis Cytosin-Arabinosid und Mitoxantron (HAM) in der Therapie bei refraktären akuten Leukämien und Morbus Hodgkin: Eine Übersicht über vier multizentrische Phase-II-Studien

W. Hiddemann[a], G. Maschmeyer[b], M. Pfreundschuh[c], W. D. Ludwig[d], K. H. Pflüger[e], N. Schmitz[f], K. Schumacher[g], E. Lengfelder[h], M. Planker[i], M. Freund[k], A. D. Ho[l], R. Donhuijsen-Ant[m], Th. Wagner[n], Th. Büchner[a]

[a] Medizinische Universitätsklinik Münster; [b] Evangelisches Krankenhaus Essen-Werden; [c] Medizinische Universitätsklinik Köln; [d] FU Berlin, Klinikum Steglitz, Abteilung Hämatologie/Onkologie; [e] Medizinische Universitätsklinik Marburg; [f] Medizinische Universitätsklinik Kiel; [g] Robert-Bosch-Krankenhaus Stuttgart; [h] Medizinische Universitätsklinik Heidelberg-Mannheim; [i] Städtische Kliniken Krefeld; [k] Medizinische Hochschule Hannover; [l] Medizinische Universitäts-Poliklinik Heidelberg; [m] St. Johannis-Hospital Duisburg-Hamborn; [n] Medizinische Universitätsklinik Lübeck

Einleitung

Cytosin-Arabinosid (Ara-C) stellt in hoher Dosierung zweifellos die derzeit wichtigste Einzelsubstanz in der Therapie akuter Leukämien dar und hat breite Anwendung sowohl in der Primärbehandlung als auch zur Therapie des Rezidivs gefunden. Dabei wurde die von Herzig et al. inaugurierte 6-tägige Monotherapie mit 12 Gaben von 3,0 g/m^2 HD Ara-C [1] in zahlreichen Studien sowohl im Hinblick auf die Dauer, die Dosis, als auch die Applikationsweise modifiziert und durch Kombinationen mit Anthrazyklinen, m-AMSA, VP-16 oder Asparaginase ergänzt. In-vitro-Untersuchungen mehrerer Arbeitsgruppen [2–5] und erste klinische Studien ließen erkennen, daß insbesondere durch die Kombination von HD Ara-C mit Mitoxantron eine Steigerung der antileukämischen Wirksamkeit ohne wesentliche Zunahme von Nebenwirkungen zu erzielen ist [6].

Auf dieser Grundlage und der für beide Substanzen nachgewiesenen Effektivität bei rezidivierter akuter myeloischer und lymphatischer Leukämie wurde die Kombination von HD-ARA-C und Mitoxantron (HAM) im Rahmen der multizentrischen Leukämie-Studiengruppen in einer Phase-II-Studie bei refraktärer akuter myeloischer Leukämie und nachfolgend bei akuter lymphatischer Leukämie im Frührezidiv oder bei primärer Therapieresistenz eingesetzt. In Fortentwicklung dieses Konzeptes wurde eine sequentielle Applikationsform (S-HAM) erarbeitet und im Rezidiv bei AML und ALL erprobt [7]. Darüber hinaus kam das HAM-Protokoll auch bei Patienten mit refraktärem oder rezidiviertem Morbus Hodgkin in einer Phase-I/II-Studie zur Anwendung.

Patienten, Therapieprotokolle und Methoden

Die im folgenden dargestellten Therapiestudien wurden an insgesamt 117 Patienten mit refraktärer oder rezidivierter AML (n = 75), ALL (n = 25) bzw. Morbus Hodgkin (n = 17) durchgeführt. Alle Patienten waren nach standardisierten Behandlungskonzepten im Rahmen der entsprechenden multizentrischen Therapiestudien vorbehandelt.

Entscheidendes Einschlußkriterium war ferner eine Wahrscheinlichkeit von weniger als 30%, mit konventionellen Maßnahmen eine erneute Remission zu erzielen, und damit eine Therapierefraktärität gegenüber herkömmlichen Behandlungsregimen [8]. Diese wurden im einzelnen wie folgt definiert:

AML

- Persistierende Blastenpopulation nach zwei Kursen der Induktionstherapie mit TAD9;
- Frührezidive mit einer Remissionsdauer von weniger als sechs Monaten;
- Später auftretende Rezidive mit persistierender Blastenpopulation nach einem erneuten TAD9-Kurs;
- Zweite und folgende Rezidive.

ALL

- Persistierende Blastenpopulation nach dem Induktionsprotokoll der BMFT-Studien;
- Rezidiv mit persistierender Blastenpopulation nach einem konventionellen Rezidivprotokoll;
- Zweite und folgende Rezidive.

Morbus Hodgkin

- Persistierende Erkrankung nach Chemo-Induktionstherapie im Stadium III B–IV B;
- Frührezidive im Stadium III B–IV mit einer Remissionsdauer von weniger als 12 Monaten;
- Spätrezidive mit persistierender Erkrankung nach konventionellen Rezidivprotokollen.

Das ursprüngliche Protokoll zur Behandlung von AML und ALL bestand aus HD-Ara-C 3 g/m^2 alle 12 h als 3-h-Infusion an den Tagen 1–4 und Mitoxantron 10 mg/m^2/Tag Tag 2–6 [6]. Im Rahmen dieser 1987 abgeschlossenen Studie wurden insgesamt 84 Patienten mit AML (n = 65) bzw. ALL (n = 19) behandelt.

In der 1987 begonnenen Anschlußstudie kam folgendes, nach pharmakokinetischen und zellkinetischen Gesichtspunkten modifiziertes Protokoll zum Einsatz [7]: HD Ara-C 3 g/m^2 alle 12 h als 3-h Dauerinfusion Tag 1 und 2, Mitoxantron 10 mg/m^2/Tag Tag 3 und 4. Nach dreitägiger Pause wurde die identische Sequenz an den Tagen 8 und 9 (HD Ara-C) bzw. 10 und 11 (Mitoxantron) wiederholt.

Die ebenfalls 1987 begonnene Phase-I/II-Studie zur Behandlung von Patienten mit refraktärem oder rezidiviertem Morbus Hodgkin bestand aus einer verkürzten Version des ursprünglichen HAM-Protokolls mit der Möglichkeit der Eskalation bei tolerabler Toxizität entsprechend dem folgenden Schema: In der ersten Stufe wurde HD Ara-C 3 g/m^2 alle 12 h als 3-h Infusion an den Tagen 1 und 2 und Mitoxantron 10 mg/m^2/Tag an den Tagen 3–5 gegeben. Bei gleichbleibender Mitoxantron-Applikation wurde HD Ara-C in Stufe 2 auf 3 Tage (6 Dosen) erweitert. Stufe 3 bestand aus jeweils vier Therapietagen von HD Ara-C (Tag 1–4 8 Dosen) und Mitoxantron (Tag 2–5).

Bei allen Protokollen erhielten die Patienten während der HD Ara-C-Applikation Glukokortikoid-Augentropfen zur Prophylaxe konjunktivaler Reizerscheinungen. Darüber hinaus wurde eine begleitende antiemetische Therapie nach Maßgabe des jeweiligen Zentrums durchgeführt. Die Beurteilung der Schwere und Dauer von Nebenwirkungen erfolgte nach den Definitionen der WHO. Die antileukämische bzw. anti-Hodgkin-Effektivität der Behandlung wurde nach etablierten Kriterien analog den entsprechenden Definitionen der Primärtherapie-Protokolle ausgewertet.

Als Dauer der kritischen Zytopenie galt die Zeit zwischen Therapiebeginn und dem posttherapeutischen Überschreiten einer Granulozytenzahl um 500/cmm bzw. Thrombozytenzahl von 20 000/cmm.

Ergebnisse

HAM bei refraktärer AML

65 Patienten mit refraktärer AML im Alter zwischen 18 und 67 Jahren wurden nach dem ursprünglichen HAM-Protokoll behandelt. 61 Patienten erhielten einen einzigen Therapiekurs, während in 4 Fällen ein zweiter, identischer Behandlungszyklus angeschlossen wurde. 35 Patienten (54%) kamen in eine komplette Remission, 2 Patienten erfüllten die Kriterien einer partiellen Remission. 16 Patienten verstarben innerhalb der ersten 6 Wochen nach Therapiebeginn und wurden als Frühtodesfälle klassifiziert. In 12 Fällen bestand eine persistierende oder nach Aplasie wieder regenerierende leukämische Blastenpopulation.

Die Zeit der kritischen Zytopenie betrug für Patienten mit kompletter oder partieller Remission im Median 28 Tage, die Zeit bis zum Erreichen der kompletten Remission lag im Median bei 36 Tagen. Die Remission dauerte im Median 4,5 Monate bei einer medianen Überlebenszeit von neun Monaten.

HAM bei refraktärer ALL

Die 19 Patienten mit refraktärer ALL, die nach dem ursprünglichen HAM-Protokoll behandelt wurden, waren zwischen 16 und 67 Jahren alt. In zwei Fällen wurde prätherapeutisch ein Philadelphia-Chromosom nachgewiesen, zwei weitere Patienten wiesen zum Zeitpunkt des Rezidivs eine ZNS-Beteiligung auf.

16 Patienten erhielten einen und 3 weitere Patienten zwei Therapiekurse.

Komplette Remissionen wurden in 9 Fällen (47%) erzielt, eine partielle Remission erreichten 2 Patienten. 5 Patienten verstarben innerhalb der ersten 6 Wochen. In drei Fällen erwies sich die ALL als therapierefraktär.

Die Dauer der kritischen Zytopenie betrug wie bei AML im Median 27 Tage, die Kriterien der kompletten Remission waren nach 33 Tagen erfüllt. Die mediane Remissionsdauer war 4 Monate, die Überlebenszeit 5,5 Monate.

S-HAM bei refraktärer AML und ALL

In die S-HAM Pilotstudie gingen 10 Patienten mit AML und 6 Patienten mit ALL ein. Alle Patienten erfüllten die Eingangskriterien der Refraktärität gegenüber konventionellen Therapiemaßnahmen. Zusätzlich waren 8 dieser Patienten mit dem ursprünglichen HAM-Protokoll vorbehandelt und befanden sich im Rezidiv nach vorausgegangener erfolgreicher HAM-Behandlung.

Von den insgesamt 16 Patienten erreichten 10 (63%) eine komplette Remission, davon 6 der 8 Patienten mit vorausgegangener Behandlung nach dem ursprünglichen HAM-Regime. Je 3 Patienten waren therapieresistent bzw. verstarben innerhalb der ersten 6 Wochen nach Behandlungsbeginn.

Die Dauer der kritischen Zytopenie betrug im Median 34 Tage, die Zeit bis zum Erreichen der Vollremission lag bei 42 Tagen. Die mediane Remissionsdauer war 3,5 Monate, die mediane Überlebenszeit 4,5 Monate.

HAM bei refraktärem Morbus Hodgkin

Die 17 im Rahmen der Phase-I/II-Studie behandelten Patienten mit refraktärem Morbus Hodgkin waren zwischen 17 und 46 Jahren alt und hatten vor HAM zwischen 2 und 4 alternative zytostatische Regime nach Versagen der Primärtherapie erhalten. Eine komplette Remission wurde bei einem Patienten erzielt, in 11 weiteren Fällen konnte eine partielle Remission erreicht werden. 1 Patient verstarb an septischen Komplikationen in Aplasie, 4 Fälle waren therapierefraktär. Die Zeit der kritischen Zytopenie betrug im Median 24 Tage.

Nebenwirkungen der HAM-Therapie

Die anteilmäßig überwiegenden Nebenwirkungen der Therapie mit HAM und S-HAM bestanden unabhängig von der Primärdiagnose in schwerer Myelosuppression (95%), Übelkeit und Erbrechen (85%), gefolgt von Durchfall (77%) und Schleimhauttoxizität (63%). Mit Ausnahme der Myelosuppression wurden Toxizitätsgrade von III und IV nach WHO-Definition jedoch bei weniger als 17% der Fälle registriert. Kardiale Komplikationen in Form von Rhythmusstörungen, Herzinsuffizienz bzw. Kardiomyopathie traten in 13% der Therapiekurse auf, dabei zweimal mit tödlichem Ausgang. 7% der Behandlungszyklen waren mit zentral-nervösen Nebenwirkungen verbunden in Form von reversiblen Sprachstörungen, Ataxie, Bewußtseinstrübung, Gleichgewichtsstörungen und in einem Fall einem letal endenden zentralen Koma.

Diskussion

Ausgehend von den dokumentierten Monoaktivitäten von HD Ara-C und Mitoxantron bei intensiv vorbehandelten Patienten mit akuten Leukämien, Hodgkin- und Non-Hodgkin-Lymphomen [9–14] wurde die Effektivität und Toxizität der Kombination beider Substanzen im Rahmen von 4 konsekutiven Phase-II-Studien bei Patienten mit fortgeschrittenen akuten Leukämien bzw. Morbus Hodgkin geprüft. In allen Fällen waren konventionelle Behandlungsmaßnahmen weitgehend ausgeschöpft und die Kriterien der Therapierefraktärität definiert durch eine Remissionswahrscheinlichkeit von weniger als 30% erfüllt [7]. Unter Berücksichtigung dieser Voraussetzungen waren die mit dem ursprünglich konzipiertem HAM-Protokoll [6] bei Patienten mit refraktärer AML und ALL erzielten Remissionsraten von 54% bzw. 47% ein eindeutiger Beleg für die hohe antileukämische Effektivität der Kombination und führten zur nachfolgenden Anwendung in der Primärtherapie bei beiden Erkrankungen.

In dem Bemühen, die antileukämische Wirksamkeit weiter zu steigern und die Nebenwirkungsrate zu senken, wurde aufgrund pharmakokinetischer und zellkinetischer Untersuchungen das Konzept der sequentiellen Applikation des HAM-Regimes (S-HAM) in Anlehnung an die von Capizzi et al. inaugurierte sequentielle Anwendung von HD Ara-C und Asparaginase entwickelt [15]. Neben der hohen Remissionsrate von 63%, die bei 16 Patienten im Rahmen der S-HAM Pilotstudie erreicht werden konnte, war vor allem bemerkenswert, daß von 8 Patienten, die im vorausgegangenen Rezidiv das ursprüngliche HAM-Protokoll erhalten hatten, 6 nach S-HAM erneut in eine Remission kamen. Diese dauerte bei 2 Patienten deutlich länger an als nach der ersten HAM-Rezidivtherapie. Erwartungsgemäß war die Zeit der kritischen Zytopenie nach S-HAM verlängert, jedoch nur um die Zeitspanne, die durch die Ausdehnung der Therapiedauer von 6 auf 11 Tage bedingt war. So waren 500 Granulozyten/cm^3 bzw. 20 000 Thrombozyten/cmm^3 nach S-HAM im Median nach 34 Tagen überschritten, im Vergleich zu 28 Tagen nach dem ursprünglichen HAM-Protokoll. Nicht-hämatologische Nebenwirkungen, in erster Linie gastrointestinale und zentralnervöse Begleiterscheinungen, waren tendenziell weniger häufig und stark ausgeprägt.

Stimuliert durch diese Ergebnisse ist das S-HAM Protokoll Grundlage einer im November 1987 initiierten multizentrischen Therapiestudie, die die Effektivität und Toxizität unterschiedlicher Dosen von HD Ara-C randomisiert vergleicht. Dabei erhalten Patienten im Alter unter 60 Jahren entweder 3,0 oder 1,0 g/m^2 HD Ara-C während bei älteren Patienten 1,0 g/m^2 HD Ara-C eingesetzt werden.

Im Vergleich zu den Resultaten der HAM-Regime bei akuten Leukämien sind die bei Patienten mit fortgeschrittenem Morbus Hodgkin vorliegenden Ergebnisse noch preliminär und bedürfen der Bestätigung und detaillierten Auswertung. Eine Ansprechrate von insgesamt 70% bei 17 intensiv vorbehandelten Patienten unterstreicht jedoch bereits die eindeutige Aktivität der HAM-Kombination auch bei dieser Erkrankung, die auch bei Non-Hodgkin-Lymphonen eine offensichtliche Wirksamkeit besitzt [16].

Insgesamt kann daher die Kombination von HD Ara-C und Mitoxantron als wirksame Therapie bei akuten Leukämien, Morbus Hodgkin und Non-Hodgkin-Lymphomen angesehen werden. Diese ist auch bei Patienten nach weitgehender Ausschöpfung konventioneller Behandlungsregime noch effektiv und erweitert das therapeutische Spektrum bei diesen Erkrankungen daher wesentlich.

Literatur

1 Herzig, R.H.; Wolff, S.N.; Lazarus, H.M.; Phillips, G.L.; Karanes, C.; Herzig, G.P.: High-dose cytosine arabinoside therapy for refractory leukemia. Blood *62:* 361–369 (1983).

2 Fountzillas, G.; Ohnuma, T.; Okano, T.; Greenspan, E.M.; Holland, J.F.: Schedule-dependent synergism of cytosine arabinoside (ARA-C) with mitoxantrone in human acute myelogenous leukemia cell line HL-60. Proc. Am. Soc. clin. Oncol. *2:* 179 (1983).

3 Wang, L.M.; Capizzi, R.L.; Contento, M.; Dimling, J.: Pharmacologic synergy between high dose Ara-C (HiDAC) and mitoxantrone (Mit) in murine leukemia L5178Y. Proc. Am. Ass. Cancer Res. *27:* 276 (1986).

4 Heinemann, V.; Murray, D.; Adams, T.; Walters, R.; Meyn, R.; Plunkett, W.: Mitoxantrone-induced DNA damage in leukemic cells is enhanced by treatment with high-dose arabinosyl-cytosine (HD Ara-C). Proc. Am. Soc. clin. Oncol. *6:* 30 (1987).

5 Hiddemann, W.; Krehmeier, C.; Zühlsdorf, M.; Wörmann, B.; Büchner, Th.: Assessment of timing and sequencing of cytosine arabinoside and mitoxantrone in acute leukemia – results of in vitro studies. Blood *72:* Suppl. 1, S. 204a (1988).

6 Hiddemann, W.; Kreutzmann, H.; Straif, K.; Ludwig, W.D.; Mertelsmann, R.; Donhuijsen-Ant, R.; Lengfelder, E.; Arlin, Z.; Büchner, Th.: High-dose cytosine arabinoside and mitoxantrone: A highly effective regimen in refractory acute myeloid leukemia. Blood *69:* 744–749 (1987).

7 Hiddemann, W.; Büchner, Th.; Essink, M.; Koch, P.; Stenzinger, W.; van de Loo, J.: High-dose cytosine arabinoside and mitoxantrone: Preliminary results of a pilot study with sequential application (S-Ham) indicating a high antileukemic activity in refractory acute leukemias. Onkologie *11:* 10–12 (1988).

8 Hiddemann, W.; Büchner, Th.; van de Loo, J.: Grundlagen der Rezidivtherapie bei akuter myeloischer Leukämie. Dt. Med. Wschr. (im Druck).

9 Kantarjian, H.; Barlogie, B.; Plunkett, W.; Velasquez, W.; McLaughin, P.; Riggs, S.; Cabanillas, F.: High-dose cytosine arabinoside in non-Hodgkin's lymphoma. J. clin. Oncol. *1:* 689–694 (1983).

10 Barnett, R.M.J.; Waxman, J.H.; Rohatiner, A.Z. S.; Dhaliwai, H.S; Gallagher, C.J.; Lister, A.T.: The use of high-dose cytosine arabinoside for non-Hodgkin's lymphoma. Semin. Oncol. *12:* Suppl. 3, S. 233–226 (1985).

11 Adelstein, D.J.; Lazarus, H.M.; Hines, J.D.; Herzig, G.P.: High-dose cytosine arabinoside in previously treated patients with poor-prognosis non-Hodgkin's lymphoma. Cancer *56:* 1493–1496 (1985).

12 Paciucci, P.A.; Cuttner, J.; Holland, J.F.: Mitoxantrone as a single agent and in combination chemotherapy in patients with refractory acute leukemia. Semin. Oncol. *11:* Suppl. 1, S. 36–40 (1984).

13 Gams, R.A.; Bryan, S.; Dukart, G.; Weiss, A.; Case, D.; Jones, S.; Stein, R.: Mitoxantrone in malignant lymphoma. Invest. New Drugs *3:* 219–222 (1985).

14 Ho, A.D.; Dörken, B.; Hunstein, W.: Mitoxantrone Monotherapie und in Kombination mit Cytosin-Arabinosid bei refraktären Hodgkin- und non-Hodgkin-Lymphomen. Cancer Res. clin. Oncol. *111:* Suppl., S. 105 (1986).

15 Capizzi, R.L.; Poole, M.; Cooper, M.R.; Richards, II, F.; Stuart, J.J.; Jackson, D.V.; White, D.R.; Spurr, C.L.; Hopkins, J.O.; Muss, H.B.; Rudnick, S.A.; Wells, R.; Gabriel,

D.; Ross, D.: Treatment of poor risk acute leukemia with sequential highdose ARA-C and asparaginase. Blood *63:* 694–700 (1984).
16 Ho, A.D.; Del Valle, F.; Hiddemann, W.; Engelhard, M.; Rückle, R.; Gerhartz, H.H.; Schlimock, G.; Thiel, E.: Treatment of refractory and relapsed non-Hodgkin lymphoma with mitoxantrone and high-dose cytarabine. Onkologie (im Druck).

Prof. Dr. W. Hiddemann, Westfälische Wilhelms-Universität,
Medizinische Klinik und Poliklinik, Abt. A,
Albert-Schweizer-Straße 33, D-4400 Münster (BRD)

Beitr Onkol, vol. 36, pp. 80–87 (Karger, Basel 1989)

Mitoxantron in Kombination mit hochdosiertem Cytosin-Arabinosid bei therapierefraktären malignen Lymphomen

J. Ollech-Chwoyka, W. Gassmann, N. Schmitz, H. Löffler

II. Medizinische Klinik und Poliklinik der Christian-Albrechts-Universität im Städtischen Krankenhaus Kiel

Einleitung

Die Primärtherapie sowohl des Morbus Hodgkin als auch der malignen Non-Hodgkin-Lymphome erfolgt in der Regel unter kurativer Zielsetzung und ist weitgehend standardisiert [1–5]; dennoch verbleiben je nach Lymphomentität und -stadium unterschiedlich hohe Prozentsätze von primär oder sekundär refraktären Erkrankungen [1, 2, 6–8], die einer Rezidivtherapie bedürfen. Kennzeichnend für die zahlreichen Rezidivtherapieregime ist [1, 9–12], daß sie in ca. einem Drittel aller Fälle eine Remission induzieren können [2], was durch eine autologe Knochenmarktransplantation auf ca. 50% komplette Remissionen gesteigert werden kann [1, 13–18]. Ho et al. leiteten eine Studie ein mit einer Kombination von Cytosin-Arabinosid und Mitoxantron in drei Eskalationsstufen, deren vorläufige Ergebnisse eine Wirksamkeit dieser Therapie bei refraktären Lymphomen belegen [19], und es ergibt sich die Fragestellung, ob durch eine weitere Eskalation der Dosen für Cytosin-Arabinosid und Mitoxantron, wie sie aus der Behandlung der akuten Leukämien bekannt ist [20–23], eine Verbesserung der Therapieergebnisse bei rekraktären malignen Lymphomen zu erreichen ist.

Patienten und Methoden

Eingangsvoraussetzungen unserer Pilotstudie waren
- Einverständnis des Patienten,
- meßbare Tumorparameter,
- primäre oder sekundäre Resistenz auf mindestens zwei etablierte Firstline-Chemotherapieregime,

- normale Leber- und Nierenfunktion,
- keine kardiopulmonale Insuffizienz,
- Karnofsky-Index ≧40% <Alter ≧18 Jahre,
- Substituierbarkeit für Thrombozyten und Erythrozyten.

Das Therapieregime (Tab. 1) sieht die Gabe von Cytosin-Arabinosid 3 g/m² i.v. als 3-h-Infusion alle 12 h an den Tagen 1–4 vor sowie die Applikation von Mitoxantron 10 mg/m² i.v. als 30-min-Kurzinfusion abends Tag 3–5 vor der Gabe von Cytosin-Arabinosid.

Intensive Konjunktivitisprophylaxe mittels Augenspülungen mit Isogutt-Augentropflösung alle 2 h Tag 1–5, hochdosierte antiemetische Therapie (Alizaprid, Metoclopramid), ausreichende Hydratation (mindestens 2,5 l Flüssigkeit pro Tag), Darmdekontamination (Co-Trimoxazol), Soorvorbeugung mittels oraler Gaben von Amphotericin B, Applikation von Allopurinol, konsequente Mundhygiene und Mundspülungen waren für alle Patienten obligatorisch vorgeschrieben.

Nach Abfall der Granulozyten unter 500/μl wurden alle Probanden einer inversen Isolation unterzogen und bei Auftreten von septischen Temperaturen erfolgte die Therapie in allen Fällen gemäß dem Studienprotokoll zur Interventionstherapie von Infektionen bei abwehrgeschwächten Patienten der Paul-Ehrlich-Gesellschaft (PEG-Protokoll) [24].

Die Bestimmung des Therapieerfolges wurde jeweils nach Wiedereinsetzen der Hämatopoese durchgeführt. Eine Therapiewiederholung erfolgt nach einem therapiefreien Intervall von mindestens vier Wochen nach Wiedereinsetzen der Hämatopoese.

Definition des Therapieerfolges war

– Komplette Remission (CR): Vollständiges Verschwinden aller objektivierbaren Krankheitserscheinungen für mindestens vier Wochen.

– Partielle Remission (PR): Reduktion der meßbaren Tumorparameter um mindestens 50% für mindestens vier Wochen.

– No change (NC): Reduktion der Tumorparameter um Werte <50% beziehungsweise Größenzunahme <25%.

– Progressive disease (PD): Größenzunahme der Tumorparameter um mehr als 25% beziehungsweise Auftreten von Neumanifestation.

Tumorparameter: Lymphknotendurchmesser in zwei Ebenen, prozentuale Knochenmarkinfiltration im histologischen Präparat [25]. Der Grad der Toxizität wurde gemäß der WHO-Definition gemessen [25].

Die Ergebnisse wurden, soweit notwendig, durch verteilungsunabhängige statistische Verfahren beschrieben (Median, Wilcox-U-Test, Mann-Whitney). Mittelwert mit Standardabweichung wurde berechnet nach Prüfung auf geringe Abweichung von einer Normalverteilung. Die statistische Auswertung wurde zum Teil in Anlehnung an das SPSS-Programm durchgeführt [32].

Tabelle 1. HAM-Regime

Cytosin-Arabinosid:	Tag 1–4 3 g/m² alle 12 h über 3 h
Mitoxantron:	Tag 3–5 10 mg/m² abends vor Ara-C über 30 min

Cave: Konjunktivitätsprophylaxe Tag 1–5; Intensive antiemetische Therapie; Darmdekontamination, Soorprophylaxe

Tabelle 2. Patienten

Patient	Geschlecht	Alter (Jahre)	Diagnose	Stadium	Erkrankungs-dauer (Jahre)	Vortherapien Remessionsgrad
E.B.	♀	21	HD(mixed)	IV B (Pulmo)	1	COPP/ABVD 1,5 ×, PD IM VP 16 1 ×, PD
R.V.	♀	28	HD (ns)	II B (Hals, Mediastinum)	3	COPP 6 × + RT, CR ABVD 6 ×, XRT, CEP 3 ×, PR
A.B.	♀	44	HD (ns)	III B	2	ABVD 5 ×, CR COPP 3 ×, PD TNI, CR; CEP 1 ×, PD
B.J.	♀	39	HD (ns)	III B	1/4	COPP/ABVD/IMEP 1 ×, PD
U.B.	♂	40	HD (ld)	III BES	1/2	ABVD/COPP/ABVD, PD, IMVP16, PD

Ergebnisse

Insgesamt wurden 13 Patienten in die Studie aufgenommen, fünf mit Morbus Hodgkin und acht mit malignem Non-Hodgkin-Lymphom (Tab. 2 und 3). In der Hodgkin-Gruppe hatten alle Probanden zumindest COPP/ABVD als Vortherapie erhalten, das Alter betrug 21–44 Jahre, der Karnofsky-Index im Mittel 60% (r 40–80), die Geschlechtsverteilung vier Frauen, ein Mann, die Anzahl der Vortherapien im Mittel n = 7 (r 3–15) und die mittlere Krankheitsdauer betrug 1 Jahr (r 1/4–3 Jahre) (Tab. 2).

Bei den Probanden mit malignem Non-Hodgkin-Lymphom (6 x hochmalignes, 2 x niedrig malignes Lymphom) hatten alle zumindest zwei Vortherapien erhalten, im Mittel 6 (r 2–9), Alter 21–50 Jahre, Geschlechtsverteilung sechs Männer und zwei Frauen, Karnofsky-Index im Mittel 60% (r 40–80%) und die mittlere Krankheitsdauer betrug 1 1/4 Jahre (r 1/4–2) (Tab. 3).

Von den fünf Patienten mit Morbus Hodgkin erhielten zwei HAM einmal, drei Probanden zweimal. Wir fanden eine komplette und partielle Remission, zweimal keine Änderung und eine Progredienz.

Tabelle 3. Patienten

Patient	Geschlecht	Alter (Jahre)	Diagnose	Stadium	Erkrankungs-dauer (Jahre)	Vortherapien Remessionsgrad
E.M.	♀	33	cb/ib NHL	IV B (KM, Haut, Liquor)	2	CHOP 7 x, PR MTX, VM26, Ara-C 2 x, PR
A.H.	♂	62	cb NHL	IV B (Peritoneum)	2	XRT, CR COP-BLAM 3 x, PD IMVP16 2 x, PD
D.K.	♂	25	Ib NHL (Burkitt)	IV B (KM, Peritoneum, Leber, Darm)	3/4	A-COML A 1,5 x, PD VCR, CTX, HDMTX VP16, Ifos, 1 x, PD XRT PD
H.L.	♂	53	cc NHL	IV B (Pulmo, Haut)	2	COP 6 x, PR COPP/PROMACE 3 x, PR
P.N.	♂	44	hochmalignes B-Zell-Lymphom	IV B (KM, Leber)	1/4	COP-BLAM, 4 x, PD IMVP 16 3 x, PD
L.H.	♂	44	cb NH	IV B (KM, Leber)	1/4	COP-BLAM, 2 x, PD IMVP16 2 x, PD
R.H.	♂	24	cc NHL	IV B (KM)	2	COP-BLAM 4 x, PR IMVP 16 5 x, PR
G.P.	♀	50	ib NHL	III B	1/2	BMFTB-ALL Protokoll, COPBLAM 2 x, PD

Bei den acht Probanden mit Non-Hodgkin-Lymphomen, ein Patient wurde zweimal therapiert, wurden zwei komplette und eine partielle Remission, drei progrediente Erkrankungen und einmalig keine Änderung beobachtet. Ein Proband konnte nicht evaluiert werden wegen Frühtodes in der Knochenmarksaplasie. Insgesamt fanden wir eine Tumorresponse in fünf von 13 Fällen.

Die Toxizität betraf vor allem das Knochenmark, in 13/13 Fällen trat eine Aplasie WHO-Grad 4 auf mit einer mittleren Dauer von 20 Tagen (r 13–33 Tage), die Thrombozyten-Substitutionspflichtigkeit betrug im Mittel 22 Tage. Septische Komplikationen (WHO Grad 2–4, Pneumonie, Colitis, «fever of unknown origin») traten in 11/13 Fällen auf, drei Patienten (2 x PD, 1 x Frühtodesfall) verstarben an septischen Komplikationen. Anorexie, Nausea und Emesis (WHO-Grad 2–3, 13/13), totale Alopezie (WHO-Grad 3, 13/13), Stomatitis (WHO-Grad 1–3, 6/13), Diarrhoen (WHO-Grad 1–2,6/13) und eine chemisch induzierte Hepatitis (WHO-Grad 1–2,4/13) waren häufige Komplikationen des HAM-Regimes. Eine Kardiotoxizität (WHO-Grad 1–3) beobachteten wir nur in 2/13 Fällen trotz zum Teil intensiver Vorbehandlung mit Anthracyclinen. Bei intensiver Prophylaxe fanden wir in keinem Fall (0/13) eine Konjunktivitis. Bei 2/13 Patienten trat ein Exanthem auf.

Diskussion

Im Vergleich zu den Untersuchungen von Ho et al. [19], deren Therapiekonzept drei Eskalationsstufen für Cytosin-Arabinosid (3 g/m^2 i.v. alle 12 h für 1, 2 oder 3 Tage) bei konstanter Dosis für Mitoxantron (10 mg/m^2 i.v. Tag 2 und 3) vorsieht, lag die von uns gewählte Cytarabindosis um 33–300% und die des Mitoxantron um 50% höher. Die erhebliche Dosiseskalation unseres Protokolls führte jedoch nicht zu einer Verbesserung der Remissionsquoten bei den Non-Hodgkin-Lymphomen. Während Ho et al. bei 5/12 Probanden (42%) einen Tumorresponse verzeichnen konnten [19], fanden wir in 3/8 Fallen (38%) ein Tumoransprechen. Die Remissionsquoten des HAM-Regimes unterscheiden sich damit nicht signifikant von denen anderer «third-line»-Therapien, die im Mittel in einem Drittel der Fälle Remissionen erzielen konnten [1, 6, 26].

Beim Morbus Hodgkin ließ sich durch das hochdosierte HAM-Regime nur in 2/5 Fällen eine Remission erzielen, wobei die Interpretation des Ergebnisses durch die kleine Fallzahl limitiert wird. Aus dem Vergleich mit den Ergebnissen anderer Autoren [9, 11, 12], die bei unterschiedlichen «third-line»-Therapien Ansprechraten von 56 bis 63% beobachteten, resultiert, daß durch das aggressivere Vorgehen keine signifikante Verbesserung der Responseraten zu erzielen war.

Die Toxizität des untersuchten hochdosierten HAM-Regimes war allerdings signifikant höher als die von Ho et al. [19] beobachtete (Knochenmarksaplasiedauer 20 versus 7 Tage, drei therapieinduzierte Todesfälle versus kein Todesfall) beziehungsweise als die der «third-line» Therapien bei Morbus Hodgkin [9, 11, 12], so daß eine Wiederholung der Therapie nur nach einem prolongierten therapiefreien Intervall von ca. sechs bis acht

Wochen Dauer den Patienten zugemutet werden konnte. Erwartungsgemäß entsprach die von uns festgestellte Toxizitätsrate weitgehend den aus der Leukämiebehandlung geläufigen Werten [20, 21, 27–30].

Insgesamt belegen unsere Daten, daß die hochdosierte Kombination von Cytosin-Arabinosid und Mitoxantron sowohl bei malignen therapierefraktären Non-Hodgkin-Lymphomen als auch beim therapierefraktären Morbus Hodgkin effektiv ist. Eine Dosiseskalation des Cytosin-Arabinosid über 2 x 3 g/m^2 i.v. über 3 Tage hinaus bewirkt keine signifikante Verbesserung der Ergebnisse, verursacht aber eine gravierende und limitierende Toxizität. Für beide Lymphomenitäten ergibt sich die Problemstellung, ob durch eine niedriger dosierte Kombination von Cytosin-Arabinosid und Mitoxantron – bei verminderter Toxizität – vergleichbare Remissionsquoten zu erzielen sind und ob die von Hiddemann et al. für die refraktären akuten myeloischen Leukämien vorgeschlagene sequentielle Applikationsweise von Cytarabin und Mitoxantron bei refraktären Lymphomen eine Verbesserung der Ergebnisse bewirken kann [31].

Literatur

1 Pfreundschuh, M.; Schaadt, M.; Diehl, V.: Chemotherapie der Non-Hodgkin-Lymphome (NHL). Internist *27:* 506–524 (1986).

2 Brittinger, G.; Gyenes, T.: Maligne Non-Hodgkin-Lymphome. Med. Welt *35:* 1389–99 (1984).

3 Diehl, V.: BMFT-Studie zum Morbus Hodgkin beim Erwachsenen. Studienprotokolle HD4, HD5 und HD6.

4 Brittinger, G.: Therapie der Non-Hodgkin-Lymphome von hohem Malignitätsgrad des Erwachsenenalters (Studienprotokoll).

5 Bonnadonna, G.: Chemotherapy of malignant lymphomas. Semin. Oncol. *12:* 1–14 (1985).

6 Bonnadonna, G.; Valagussa, P.; Santoro, A.: Prognosis of bulky Hodgkin's disease threated with radiotherapy. Cancer Surv. *4:* 439–458 (1985).

7 Gobbi, P.G.; Federico, M.; Prisco, U.A.; Salingardi, V.; Cavalli, C.; Bertolini, D.; Rossi, A.; Mauri, C.; Ascari, E.: Hodgkin's disease prognosis: a directly predective equation. Lancet *i:* 675–679 (1988).

8 Loeffler, M.; Pfreundschuh, M. et al.: Prognostic risk factors in advanced Hodgkin's lymphoma. Blut *56:* 273–281 (1988).

9 Pfreundschuh, M.G.; Schoppe, W.D.; Fuchs, R.; Pflüger, K.H.; Loeffler, M.; Diehl, V.: Lomustine, etoposide, vindesine, and dexamethasone (CEVD) in Hodgkin's lymphoma refractory to cyclophosphamide, vincristine, procarbazine, and prednisolone (COPP) and doxorubicin, bleomycin, vinblastine, and dacarbazine (ABVD): a multicenter trial of the German Hodgkin Study Group. Cancer Treat. Rep. *71:* (1987).

10 Bergsagel, D.E.: Salvage treatment for Hodgkin's disease in relapse. J. clin. Oncol. *5:* 525–526 (1987).

11 Hagemeister, F.B.; Tannir, N.; McLaughlin, P.; Salvador, P.; Riggs, S.; Valesquez, W.S.; Cabanillas, F.: MIME chemotherapy (methyl-GAG, ifosfamide, methotrexate, etoposide) as treatment for recurrent Hodgkin's disease. J. clin. Oncol. *5:* 556–561 (1987).

12 Bonnadonna, G.; Vivianis, S.; Valagussa, P.; Bonfante, V.; Santoro, A.: Third-line salvage chemotherapie in Hodgkin's disease. Semin. Oncol. *12:* Suppl. 2, S. 23–25 (1985).

13 Armitage, J.; Gingrich, A.; Klassen, L.; Bieman, P.; Kugler, J.; Fyfe, M.: Salvage therapy for advanced lymphoma using high dose cytarabine, Cyclophosphamide, total body irradiation (TBI) and autologous bone marrow transplantation. Blood *62:* 210 (1983).

14 Wolff, S.N.; Philipps, G.L., Fay, J.W.: treatment of advanced Hodgkin disease with intensive chemotherapy and autologues bone marrow transplantation (ABMT). Blood *66:* 256a (1985).

15 Jagannath, S.; Armitage, J.O.; Dicke, K.A.: Autologous bone marrow transplantation (ABMT) for relapsed Hodgkin disease. Third International Conference on Malignant Lymphoma in Rom, Abstract No. 18 (1987).

16 Appelbaum, F.R.; Sullivan, K.M.; Buckner, C.D.: Treatment of malignant lymphoma im 100 patients with chemotherapy, total body irradiation, and bone marrow transplantation. J. clin. Oncol. *5:* 1340–1347 (1987).

17 Philip, T.; Biron, P.; Maganinchi, D.: Role of massive chemotherapy and ABMT in non-Hodgkin malignant lymphoma. Lancet *ii:* 391 (984).

18 Philip, T.; Armitage, J.O.; Spitzer, G.: High-dose therapy and autologous bone marrow transplantation after failure of conventional chemotherapy in adults with intermediate grade or high-grade non-Hodgkin lymphoma. New Engl. J. Med. *316:* 1493–1498 (1987).

19 Ho, A.D.; Hiddemann, W.; Thiel, E.; Hunstein, W.: Erfahrungen mit Mitoxantron in Kombination mit hochdosiertem Cytarabin bei Non-Hodgkin-Lymphomen. FAC *6–9:* 1535–1538 (1987).

20 Hiddemann, W.; Kreutzmann, H.; Straif, K.; Planker, M.; Donhuijsen-Ant, R.; Lengfelder, E.; Büchner, Th.: Behandlung refraktärer akuter Leukämien mit Mitoxantron in Kombination mit Hochdosis-Cytosin-Arabinosid (HAM). FAC *6–9:* 1505–1510 (1987).

21 Fuchs, H.G.; Kolbe, K.; Herrmann, F.; Mertelsmann, R.: Vorläufige Ergebnisse der Kombination Hochdosis-Cytosin-Arabinosid und Mitoxantron (HAM) bei Patienten mit akuter myeloischer Leukämie in der Sekundär- und Primärbehandlung. FAC *6–9:* 1511–1515 (1987).

22 Hoelzer, D.; Buechner, Th.; Freund, M.; Ganser, A.; Heil, G.; Hiddemann, W.; Löffler, H.; Maschmeyer, G.; Messerer, D.; Thiel, E.: Multizentrische intensivierte Therapiestudie: Akute lymphathische und akute undifferenzierte Leukämie des Erwachsenen (Studienprotokoll) (1988).

23 Büchner, Th.; Urbanitz, D.; Löffler, H.; Hossfeld, D.K.: Anschlußstudie 1985 AML des Erwachsenen (Studienprotokoll).

24 PEG-Studienprotokoll ZAC *3:* (1985).

25 Miller, A.B.; Hoogstraten, B.; Staquet, M.; Winkler, A.: Reporting results of cancer treatment. Cancer *47:* 207–214 (1981).

26 Meuserus, P.; Zou, P.; Dührsen, U.; Brittinger, G.: Die Therapie des refraktären Non-Hodgkin-Lymphoms (NHL). Tumor Diagn. Therap. *6:* 87–91 (1986).

27 Kuse, R.; Küchler, K.: Nicht-hämatologische Toxizität bei der hochdosierten Cytarabin-Therapie. Onkologie *8:* 20–22 (1985).

28 Jahn, U.: Erfahrungen mit der HD-Ara-C-Behandlung bei Leukämie-Patienten. Onkologie *8:* 37–38 (1985).

29 Brudler, O.; Heil, G.; Kurrle, E.: Hochdosis Cytosin-Arabinosid in der Behandlung rezidivierter oder refraktärer akuter myeloischer Leukämien. Onkologie *8:* 39–43 (1985).

30 Nowrousian, M.R.; Seeber, S.; Miller, A.A.; Anders, Ch.; Öhl, S.; Schmidt, C.G.: Hochdosierte Cytarabin-Behandlung bei akuten Leukämien und Meningiosis leucaemica: Klinik und Pharmakokinetik. Onkologie *8:* 26–32 (1985).

31 Hiddemann, W.; Büchner, Th.: Prospektive randomisierte Studie zur Behandlung der akuten myeloischen Leukämie des Erwachsenen im Rezidiv und bei primärer Therapieresistenz: Vergleich von hochdosiertem und mittel hochdosiertem Cytosin-Arabinosid in Kombination mit Mitoxantrone und nachfolgender prolongierter Konsolidisierungsbehandlung (Studienprotokoll) (1987).

32 Nie, W.H.; Hull, C.H.; Jenkins, J.C.; Steinbrenner, K.; Bent, D.H.: SPSS: Statistical Package for the Social Sciences. (McGraw, New York 1975).

Dr. J. Ollech-Chwoyka, II. Medizinische Klinik und Poliklinik
der Christian-Albrechts-Universität Kiel im Städtischen Krankenhaus Kiel,
Metzstraße 53–57, D-2300 Kiel (BRD)

Beitr Onkol, vol. 36, pp. 88–95 (Karger, Basel 1989)

Möglichkeiten und Grenzen der Tumortherapie mit Zytokinen

F. Herrmann, A. Lindemann, R. Mertelsmann

Abteilung für Hämatologie, Johannes Gutenberg-Universität, Mainz

Die Behandlung fortgeschrittener Tumorerkrankungen ist nach wie vor eine Domäne der Chemotherapie, die jedoch vom Prinzip her relativ unspezifisch wirkt, da sie gleichermaßen auf alle rasch wachsenden Gewebe, ob gut- oder bösartig, einen zellschädigenden (zytostatischen oder zytotoxischen) Effekt ausübt. Daraus erklärt sich nicht nur das schwerwiegende Nebenwirkungsprofil, sondern letztlich auch die limitierte Effektivität der Chemotherapie. Trotz hochdifferenzierter Kombinationsschemata sind nur weniger als 5% aller disseminierten Krebserkrankungen heilbar [1].

Eine langfristige Verbesserung der Ergebnisse der Krebstherapie setzt Behandlungsformen voraus, die am pathophysiologischen Tumorverhalten oder an der Tumor-/Wirt-Interaktion orientiert sind. Bislang wird mit dem Begriff «Krebs» die Vorstellung verbunden, daß Heilung alleine durch radikale Vernichtung der Tumorzellen erreichbar sei, nicht aber durch eine Beeinflussung des Zellstoffwechsels, wie dies bei gutartigen Erkrankungen möglich ist. Forschungsergebnisse der letzten Jahre zeigten jedoch, daß auch bösartiges Wachstum Ausdruck einer Fehlsteuerung sein kann, die potentiell durch den Organismus (Wirt) oder exogen manipulierbar ist. Die Situation ist in gewisser Hinsicht vergleichbar derjenigen angeborener Stoffwechseldefekte, mit dem Unterschied, daß nicht spezifisch differenzierte Zellfunktionen betroffen sind (z. B. Enzymdefekte), sondern zentrale und allgemeine Funktionen der Wachstumsregulation. Die Folge ist vielfach eine blockierte Ausreifung, so daß die Zellen zu permanentem Wachstum gezwungen sind, ohne in den stabilen Zustand der reifen Funktionszelle zu differenzieren. Der primäre Defekt liegt zumeist auf genetischer Basis, verursacht durch unterschiedliche Agentien (Viren, ionisierende Strahlen,

Mutagene, spontan), die selbst aber im Hinblick auf die unmittelbaren Folgen für den Zellstoffwechsel von sekundärer Bedeutung sind. Das Resultat ist eine quantitativ oder qualitativ veränderte Produktion von Proteinen, die Schlüsselfunktion im Regelungssystem von Wachstum und Differenzierung einnehmen. Dazu gehören insbesondere Wachstumsfaktoren, ihre Rezeptoren, zytoplasmatische Transmittermoleküle und regulativ wirkende DNS-bindende Proteine. Da die entsprechenden Gene im Falle fehlerhafter Expression Malignität zu induzieren vermögen, werden sie als die sogenannten Proto-Onkogene bezeichnet [13].

Wenn eine Mutation mit neoplastischem Wachstum eingetreten ist, so ist diese in aller Regel von einem veränderten Muster synthetisierter Proteine (Genexpressionsmuster) begleitet. Damit ist die autonom wachsende Zellpopulation aber nicht autark, sondern nach wie vor von der intensiven Interaktion mit den physiologischen Systemen des Wirtsorganismus abhängig (z. B. Hormonabhängigkeit mancher Krebsformen). Mit seinem Immunsystem kann sich der Organismus dann gegen einen Tumor wenden, wenn infolge einer Mutation die Tumorzelle an der Membran Strukturmerkmale exprimiert, die vom tumortragenden Wirt als «fremd» erkannt werden.

Für eine diesen Gesichtspunkten Rechnung tragende Therapie ergeben sich konzeptionell drei Zugangswege zum krebskranken Patienten:

1. Stimulation des Immunsystems mit dem Ziel der Potenzierung von gegen Krebszellen gerichteten immunologischen Abwehrmaßnahmen (z. B. Interleukin 2).

2. Die Modulation von Tumorzellproliferation und Tumorzelldifferenzierungsvermögen (phänotypische Reversion) durch zytotoxische, zytostatische oder regulatorisch wirkende Substanzen (Tumor-Nekrose-Faktoren, Interferone).

3. Stimulation unspezifischer Wirtresistenz und Abschwächung von Chemotherapie bedinger Toxizität (z. B. hämatopoetische Wachstumsfaktoren).

Diese genannten Faktoren sind unter dem Oberbegriff «Zytokine» subsumiert. Es handelt sich hierbei um hormonähnliche interzelluläre Messenger-Moleküle, die physiologisch im Organismus gebildet werden, und auch unter physiologischen Bedingungen spezifisch in die Wachstumskontrolle bestimmter Zelltypen, insbesondere im Rahmen der spezifischen Immunantwort, der Entzündungsreaktion sowie auch der Regulation der Bildung hämato-/lymphopoetischer Zellen eingeschaltet sind. Der klinische Einsatz dieser in großen Mengen rekombinant herstellbarer Substanzen ist jedoch durch ein heterogenes Spektrum von Zielzellen und Wirkungen kompliziert. Die In-vivo-Effekte der Zytokine sind daher nur aproximativ voraussagbar.

Im folgenden werden die gegenwärtig verfügbaren Zytokine dargestellt, soweit sie für den Onkologen für Interesse sind.

Interferone

Bereits einen bedeutsamen Stellenwert in der Zytokin-Therapie haben die Interferone erfahren. Sie bilden zwei Gruppen von Glykoproteinen, die primär durch ihre zellschützende Wirkung gegenüber Virusinfektionen identifiziert wurden. Ein zentraler Interferon-Effekt besteht offenbar in der Hemmung zellulärer Proliferation durch Induktion des 2', 5'-Oligoadenylat-RNAse Systems oder der Einleitung von Differenzierungsvorgängen durch Suppression Proliferation-induzierender Proto-Onkogene. Dieser antiproliferative Effekt führte schließlich zum Einsatz insbesondere von alpha-Interferon in der Tumortherapie. Von dem breiten Spektrum untersuchter Tumoren erwiesen sich insbesondere die Haarzell-Leukämie (vergleiche den Beitrag von H. Pralle in diesem Band) sowie die chronische myeloische Leukämie als sensitiv. Bei einzelnen soliden Tumoren ließ sich mit alpha-Interferon ebenfalls, allerdings limitierte, Tumorregression erzielen, wie bei dem malignen Melanom, dem oberflächlichen Harnblasen-Karzinom, dem Ovarial-Karzinom und Kaposi-Sarkom [9].

Interleukin 2

Interleukin 2 ist ein zentrales Molekül für die Amplifikation und funktionelle Aktivierung immunkompetenter Lymphozyten. Sein klinischer Einsatz basiert insbesondere auf seiner Fähigkeit zur polyklonalen Amplifikation zytotoxischer Lymphozyten, insbesondere den sogenannten Lymphokin-aktivierten Killerzellen (LAK-Zellen). Die Gabe von Interleukin 2 mit zuvor in vitro durch Interleukin 2 expandierten und aktivierten autologen Killerzellen, die durch Zellseparation vom Patienten gewonnen wurden, hat in einigen amerikanischen Studien signifikante Anti-Tumoreffekte, insbesondere beim Hypernephrom und malignen Melanom, demonstriert [11, 14]. In diesen Studien wurde aufgrund proportionaler Dosiswirkungsbeziehung eine maximale tolerierbare Interleukin-2-Dosis mit zum Teil schwerwiegenden Nebenwirkungen verabreicht, wie kardiovaskulären Komplikationen, massiver Ödembildung durch Zunahme der Gefäßpermeabilität und hierdurch bedingtem Albuminverlust. Gleichwohl die Mechanismen, die zu diesem «capillary leakage syndrome» führen, noch nicht im Detail klar sind, spricht doch vieles für eine unspezifische und gegen Endothelzellen gerichtete Zytotoxizität von LAK-Zellen, die sich bisher jedoch in allen Therapien als reversibel erwiesen hat. Das Toxizitätsproblem der LAK-Behandlung hat schließlich zu Modifikationen des ursprünglichen Behandlungskonzeptes geführt. Derzeit werden zwei Konzepte verfolgt:

1. Verbesserung der Tumorspezifität der Interleukin-Behandlung.
2. Steigerung der Effektivität von Interleukin 2 durch gleichzeitige Gabe synergisierender Substanzen mit Anti-Tumoreffektivität.

In dem erstgenannten Rahmen ist sicher die klinische Verwendung von zytotoxischen T-Zellen (CTL) zu diskutieren, die in ihrer Killerpotenz diejenige von LAK-Zellen übertreffen. Gegenwärtige Bemühungen, solche CTL-Zellen zu generieren, fokussieren auf Interleukin 4 als induzierendes Zytokin und auf Interleukin-4-sensitive Zellen mit der Potenz zur Infiltration von Tumorgewebe (tumorinfiltrierende Lymphozyten; TIL-Zellen) [12]. Andere Möglichkeiten, tumoraffine T-Lymphozyten zu rekrutieren, wurden in Tiermodellen durch die lokale Administration von Interleukin 2 am Tumorort untersucht. Insbesondere in Kombination mit tumorsensibilisierten T-Zellen waren hier signifikante Anti-Tumoreffekte erzielbar [2]. Andere klinische Untersuchungen haben die Möglichkeit der Gabe synergistischer Chemotherapeutika mit Interleukin 2 untersucht, wobei insbesondere die Kombination mit niedrigdosiertem Cyclophosphamid erwähnt werden muß. Erste klinische Ergebnisse zeigten allerdings, daß auch mit diesem Vorgehen keine signifikante Tumorreduktion möglich ist [10].

Tumor-Nekrose-Faktor alpha

Bei Tumor-Nekrose-Faktor alpha handelt es sich um ein von Monozyten/Makrophagen, T-Lymphozyten, B-Lymphozyten (vergleiche den Beitrag von F. Porzsolt in diesem Band) sowie Granulozyten produziertes Molekül. Im Hinblick auf normales Gewebe ist Tumor-Nekrose-Faktor alpha ein pleiotropes Zytokin, das die Funktion einer Vielzahl von verschiedenen Organsystemen zu modulieren vermag. Fibroblasten, Chondrozyten, Osteoblasten, Osteoklasten, Hepatozyten, Muskelzellen, Endothelzellen, Synoviazellen, Gliazellen, Epithelzellen, Adipozyten, hämatopoetische

Stammzellen und hämatopoetische Endzellen wie Eosinophile, Neutrophile, T-Lymphozyten, B-Lymphozyten und natürliche Killerzellen haben sich als Tumor-Nekrose-Faktor rezeptiv und durch Tumor-Nekrose-Faktor funktionell beeinflußbar erwiesen. Insbesondere aufgrund seiner außergewöhnlichen Anti-Tumoraktivität im Tiermodell und seiner bevorzugt gegen Tumorzellen gerichteten zytotoxischen Aktivität hat Tumor-Nekrose-Faktor schließlich auch Eingang in die Krebstherapie gefunden [5]. In ersten klinischen Studien in den Vereinigten Staaten sowie Europa wurde Tumor-Nekrose-Faktor alpha bei Tumorpatienten in Einzeldosen von 1–400 mcg/m^2 Körperoberfläche/die als intravenöse oder subkutane Injektion gegeben, untersucht. Obwohl bei beiden Administrationswegen Serumspiegel identifiziert wurden, die in vitro Anti-Tumoraktivität aufwiesen, war die in vivo erzielbare Tumorreduktion höchst unbefriedigend. Etwa 5% der behandelten Patienten zeigten objektiven Tumorregreß, wobei insbesondere kolorektale Karzinome oder Hypernephrome als Zielgruppe für künftige Phase-II-Studien definiert wurden [4]. Die Tumor-Nekrose-Faktor-Behandlung weist ein ähnliches Nebenwirkungsspektrum wie dasjenige mit Interleukin 2 auf. Auch hier tritt ein «capillary leakage syndrome» als dosis-limitierende Toxizität auf. Aufgrund dieser Nebenwirkungen sind die im Menschen applizierbaren Tumor-Nekrose-Faktor-Dosen nur etwa $^1/_{50}$ der äquivalenten tumorizidalen Dosis bei der Maus. Es müssen daher weitere Untersuchungen zeigen, ob eine Dosissteigerung von Tumor-Nekrose-Faktor durch den gleichzeitigen Einsatz von nebenwirkungsabschwächenden Substanzen erreichbar ist und ob eine ähnliche Anti-Tumorwirksamkeit wie im Tiermodell auch im Menschen erzielt werden kann. In diesem Zusammenhang wäre die Kopplung von Tumor-Nekrose-Faktor an tumorreaktive Antikörper sicher von besonderem Interesse, um so bei maximaler Tumor-Nekrose-Faktor-Akkumulation am Tumorort minimale systemische Toxizität zu gewährleisten.

Granulozyten/Makrophagen-Kolonie-stimulierender Faktor

Granulozyten/Makrophagen-Kolonie-stimulierender Faktor (GM-CSF) ist ein Mitglied der Familie der hämatopoetischen Wachstumsfaktoren ([7]. Abgesehen von Erythropoietin, dessen therapeutische Effektivität in der Behandlung der renalen Anämie dokumentiert ist [3], befindet sich die In-vivo-Testung der CSFs erst im Anfangsstadium. In Tierexperimenten beim Menschenaffen konnte gezeigt werden, daß durch die Gabe von GM-CSF die Dauer einer Zytostatika- und Strahlen-induzierten Knochenmarksschädigung erheblich verkürzt werden konnte; auch die Zeitspanne bis zur Wiederausbildung eines normalen Knochenmarkes bzw. peripheren Blutbildes nach autologer Knochenmarkstransplantation konnte erheblich verkürzt werden. Derzeit sind weltweit die ersten Phase-I-Studien mit rekombinantem humanem GM-CSF bei Patienten mit AIDS, myelodysplastischen Syndrom, aplastischer Anämie, autologer Knochenmarkstransplantation und Chemotherapie-refraktärem Tumorleiden durchgeführt worden [8]. Die anfängliche Hoffnung, daß sich dieses Molekül zur Reduktion der Chemotherapie-assoziierten Knochenmarkstoxizität und somit zur Reduktion von Infektionskomplikationen bei Chemotherapie verwenden ließe, konnte nach bisher vorliegenden Ergebnissen erfüllt werden. Auch im Rahmen der autologen Knochenmarkstransplantation ist eine eindeutige Beschleunigung der Autorekonstitution erzielbar. In chemotherapeutischen Situationen, in denen die Myelotoxizität des applizierten Zytostatikums dosislimitierend ist, könnte die In-vivo-Expansion hämatopoetischer Zellen zur Dosissteigerung des entsprechenden Zytostatikums verhelfen oder die termingerechte Applikation eines chemotherapeutischen Zyklus gewährleisten. GM-CSF hat sich darüber hinaus als ein Aktivator von Granulozyten- und Monozytenfunktionen erwiesen, die normal vom Organismus auch als Instrumentarium seines tumoriziden Repertoires genutzt werden. Eine objektive Tumorrückbildung mit GM-CSF haben die bisher durchgeführten Studien jedoch nicht gezeigt. Verglichen mit anderen Zytokin-Therapieformen ist diejenige mit GM-CSF als nebenwirkungsarm einzustufen. In einer eigenen Studie [6] blieben unabhängig von Dosisstufe und Applikationsdauer und -art 35% der Patienten nebenwirkungsfrei. Grad-III-Toxizität trat bei etwa 10% der behandelten Tumorpatienten auf. Bei diesen Patienten kam es zu Atemnotzuständen während der Initialphase der Infusion, vermutlich durch rasche Sequestration von Neutrophilen im Lungenkreislauf.

Kürzliche In-vitro-Untersuchungen in Primatenmodellen haben die Möglichkeit der kombinierten Anwendung verschiedener hämatopoetischer Wachstumsfaktoren in Aussicht gestellt, wobei die synergistische Aktivität verschiedener solcher Faktoren die Rationale für ihren Einsatz in Zytokin-Kombinationen darstellt. In diesem Zusammenhang scheint insbesondere die Kombination von GM-CSF mit Interleukin 3 von Bedeutung, die eine Stimulation auch der Megakaryopoese in Aussicht stellt. Erste klinische Studien von Interleukin 3 mit GM-CSF werden in Kürze über diese Möglichkeiten Aufschlüsse geben.

Ausblick

Insgesamt sind die Ergebnisse der Therapie mit den sogenannten biologisch aktiven Substanzen gegenwärtig als unbefriedigend zu bezeichnen, da dem überwiegenden Teil von Tumorpatienten auf diese Weise bislang nicht geholfen werden konnte. Für die teilweise enttäuschenden In-vivo-Effekte eine fundierte Erklärung zu geben, hätte zur Voraussetzung, das physiologische Netzwerk interagierender Faktoren und letztlich das Phänomen neoplastischen Wachstums zu verstehen. Da der Stand der Forschung hiervon noch weit entfernt ist, bestehen diesbezüglich nur Hypothesen. Sehr wahrscheinlich spielt jedoch die Heterogenität der Tumoren eine entscheidende Rolle. Die potentiell therapeutisch beeinflußbare Zellstoffwechselstörung dürfte zumindestens für die Art des Tumors spezifisch sein, so daß eine pathogenetisch orientierte Chemotherapie jenes Wissen zur Voraussetzung hätte, das uns heute noch weitgehend fehlt. In dieser Hinsicht ist die Entdeckung der spezifischen Wirksamkeit des Interferon-alpha bei der Haarzell-Leukämie als Zufall anzusehen. Der Schwerpunkt der gegenwärtig verfügbaren Zytokine wird in der therapeutischen Beeinflussung der Tumor-/Wirt-Interaktion liegen, das heißt, nicht die direkte Anti-Tumoraktivität, sondern die Modulation der Reaktion des Wirtes auf seinen Tumor oder auf eine Chemotherapie wird im Vordergrund stehen. Weil dieser eher indirekte Effekt insbesondere für die Kolonie-stimulierenden Faktoren mit ihrer relativ gut charakterisierten physiologischen Wirkung zutrifft, dürfte ihnen unter den zur Zeit in Prüfung befindlichen Substanzen in nächster Zukunft die größte Bedeutung zukommen. Wenn es gelingt, die Knochenmarkssuppression als eine der wesentlichen und dosislimitierenden Nebenwirkungen der Chemotherapie durch den Einsatz von Kolonie-stimulierenden Faktoren wirksam zu beeinflussen, würde die Zahl lebensbedrohlicher Komplikationen, insbesondere von Infektionen, erheblich reduziert werden können.

Literatur

1 Baylar, J.C.; Smith, E.M.: Progress against cancer? New Engl. J. Med. *314:* 1226–1232 (1986).

2 Cheever, M.A.; Greenberg, P.D.; Fefer, A.: A specific adoptive therapy of established leukemia with syngeneic lymphocytes sequentially immunized in vitro and in vivo and non-specifically expanded by culture with interleukin 2. J. Immunol. *126:* 1318–1326 (1981).

3 Eschbach, J.W.; Egrie, J.C.; Downing, M.R.; Browne, J.K.; Adamson, J.W.: Correction of anemia of end-stage renal disease with recombinant human erythropoietin. New Engl. J. Med. *316:* 73–78 (1987).

4 Gamm, H.; Herrmann, F.; Flener, R.; Mull, R.; Mertelsmann, R.: Tumor necrosis factor-alpha in advanced cancer: A phase I study. Mol. Biother. (in Druck).
5 Herrmann, F.; Mertelsmann, R.: Tumor Nekrose Faktor. Dt. Med. Wschr. *114:* 312–316 (1989).
6 Herrmann, F.; Mertelsmann, R.: Polypeptides controlling hematopoietic blood cell formation and activation. I: In vitro results. Blut *58:* 117–129 (1989).
7 Herrmann, F.; Schulz, G.; Lindemann, A.; Meyenburg, W.; Oster, W.; Krumwieh, D.; Mertelsmann, R.: Yeast-expressed GM-CSF in cancer patients: A phase I b clinical study. Behring Inst. Mitt. *83:* 107–118 (1988).
8 Krumwieh, D.; Schulz, G.; Seiler, F. R.: Rationales for the development of the human hematopoietic colony stimulating factors as therapeutical useful drugs. Behring Inst. Mitt. *82:* 265–281 (1988).
9 Lindemann, A.; Oster, W.; Herrmann, F.; Mertelsmann, R.: Zytokine in der Tumortherapie. Drug. Res. *38:* 466–470 (1988).
10 Mertelsmann, R.; Lindemann, A.; Kolitz, J.; Herrmann, F.: Synergism between cyclophosphamide and interleukin-2. CRC Crit. Rev. Hematol. Oncol. (in Druck).
11 Rosenberg, S.A.: Immunotherapy of cancer using interleukin 2: Current status and future prospects. Immunol. Today *9:* 58–62 (1988).
12 Topalian, S.L.; Solomon, D.; Avis, F.P.; Chang, A.E.; Freerksen, D.C.; Linehan, H. W.; Lotze, M.T.; Robertson, C.N.; Seipp, C.A.; Simon, P.; Simpson, C.G.; Rosenberg, S.A.; Immunotherapy of patients with advanced cancer using tumor infiltrating lymphocytes and recombinant interleukin 2. J. Clin. Oncol. *6:* 839–853 (1988).
13 Vogt, P.K.: Oncogenes and signals of cell growth. Drug. Res. *37:* 243–252 (1987).
14 West, W.H.; Tauer, K.W.; Yanelli, J.R.; Marshall, G.D.; Orr, D.W.; Thurman, G.B.; Oldham, R.K.: Constant infusion of recombinant interleukin-2 in adoptive immunotherapy of cancer. New Engl. J. Med. *316:* 898–905 (1987).

Prof. Dr. F. Herrmann, Abteilung für Hämatologie, Johannes Gutenberg-Universität, Langenbeckstr. 1, D-6500 Mainz (BRD)

Beitr Onkol, vol. 36, pp. 96–105 (Karger, Basel 1989)

Interferontherapie der Haarzell-Leukämie

H. Pralle

Abteilung Hämatologie/Onkologie, Medizinische Kliniken der Justus-Liebig-Universität Gießen

Die außergewöhnlich sicher auf α-Interferon (Ifn α) ansprechende Haarzell-Leukämie (HCL) ist eine seltene Erkrankung. In der Bundesrepublik werden im Jahr etwa 120 Fälle diagnostiziert, überwiegend bei Männern im Alter von etwa 50 Jahren. Nur $^1/_6$–$^1/_4$ der Patienten wird von etwas jüngeren Frauen gestellt. Die vorwiegend in der Milz akkumulierenden Zellen werden den B-Lymphozyten zugerechnet. Sie sind in fast allen Fällen auf die Immunglobulinsynthese soweit vorbereitet, daß sie die Genabschnitte für die Immunglobuline sowohl für die Leicht- wie die Schwerketten rearrangiert haben. Dementsprechend werden Haarzellen auch als Präplasmazellen bezeichnet [1]. Ein tiefgreifender und unerklärter Defekt betrifft die Monozytopoiese [2]. Er trägt wahrscheinlich wesentlich zu den oft komplizierenden mykobakteriellen Infektionen bei. Andere Zeichen können vermehrte Faserbildung und Osteoidbildung sein. Die Infiltration von Sinusoiden der roten Pulpa der Milz und dem Knochenmark sowie an Basalmembranen von Lunge, Peritoneum und anderen Organen scheinen die Clearancefunktion für alle Mikroben zu beeinträchtigen. So starben bisher 80% der Patienten an Infektionen nach einer medianen Lebenswahrscheinlichkeit von etwa 6 Jahren [3]. Diese Infektionen spielen schon zu Beginn der Erkrankung eine große Rolle. Bis in letzte Zeit erreichen viele Patienten mit HCL die Diagnose und damit ihre Therapiemöglichkeit erst, wenn die verschiedensten Infektionen mit oft atypischen Verläufen ein klassisches Bild ergeben haben, die den Patienten zu Therapiebeginn zusätzlich gefährden.

Die Wirkung von α-Ifn auf die HCL ist 5 Jahre nach ihrer Entdeckung durch Quesada [4] unter drei verschiedenen Gesichtspunkten zu diskutieren und für die beiden Behandlungsphasen Remissionserzeugung und -erhaltung zu beschreiben.

Zur Anwendungsweise und Effizienz in der Anfangstherapie:

1. Über den Beginn der Therapie mit α-Ifn ist oft berichtet worden. α-Ifn zeigt dabei sehr komplexe Wirkungen und Nebenwirkungen. Neben den kurzfristigen sind heute auch schon mittelfristige Ergebnisse bekannt, die zunehmend sicherer erlauben werden, den Wert der α-Ifn-Therapie gegenüber der konventionellen Behandlung abzuschätzen. Ein Platz auf der Therapieleiter für eine langverlaufende Erkrankung ist abzusehen. Deshalb werden hier die Daten zur Anwendung von α-Ifn aus den großen Studien zur HCL global dargestellt (Tab. 1) und nur ausführlicher diskutiert.

2. Bei der Anwendung von α-Ifn ergaben sich Lerneffekte für die Nomenklatur zu biologischen Substanzen und ihrer Wirkungen. Man mußte den Aspekt des negativ wirkenden Zytokins beim Umgang mit schwerkranken Patienten mehr berücksichtigen. Der erstgewählte Ausdruck Immunmodulator konnte nicht mit Gehalt gefüllt werden [5]. Noch weniger ist der Ausdruck «biological response modifier» (BRM) zu fassen gewesen.

Tabelle 1. Therapieergebnisse, die mit verschiedenen Typ I-Interferonen bei der Haarzellen-Leukämie erzielt wurden (Auswahl)

	Dosis $\times 10^6$ U	Wiederholung	Gabe		Patientenzahl (evaluiert)	Ergebnis CR	PR	MR	NR	Autor	
Natürlich											
leu	3	tgl	s. c.		22	5	13	4	0	Quesada	[4]
leu	3	tgl (5/28)	s. c.		6	2	3	1	0	Clark	[8]
n_1	2/m²	3/Wo				2	7	2	2	Glaspy	[25]
n_1	3	tgl	i.m.,s.c.		17	2	13	2	0	Worman	[11]
fibro	50	3/Wo	i.v.		8	0	3	2	3	v. Wussow	[12]
Gemischt											
leu	3	tgl	s.c.	25	27	2	8	14	0	Castaigne	[16]
n_1	3	tgl		9							
2b	2/m²	3/Wo		19							
Rekombinant											
2a	3-(12)	tgl	s.c.		30	5	17	6	2	Quesada	[9]
2b	2/m²	3/Wo	s.c.		128	4	98	9	16	Golomb	[10]
					85	3	59	14	5	Schwarzmeier	[24]
2c	1,2/m²	tgl × 84	s.c.	81/	73	2	36	33	2	Pralle	[15]
Rekombinant β											
β ser	50	tgl × 14/28	i.v.		7	0	5	2	0	Glaspy	[25]

Die beiden letzten Begriffe werden deshalb ohne weitere Erkenntnisse besser nicht verwendet. Der Remissionsbegriff mußte mit neuen Zeitvorgaben ergänzt werden. So wurden während der Therapiebeobachtungen neue Definitionen für biologisch wirksame Protokolle entwickelt. Die optimal biologisch aktive Ifn-Therapie konnte der maximal tolerierten Chemotherapie komplementär entgegengesetzt werden.

3. Unter den neuen Entwicklungen im Umfeld der Ifn-Therapie wurde schon die Nachfolgebehandlung erkennbar. Fast gleichzeitig mit der Einführung des α-Ifns erschienen medikamentöse Alternativen: Deoxicoformycin beeinflußt offenbar manche Lymphozytenpopulationen so günstig, daß einige Patienten mit HCL und mit Immunozytomen mit langanhaltenden Remissionen rechnen können [6] und Wachstumsfaktoren der Hämopoiese erreichen jetzt die klinische Versuchsphase [7]. Damit könnten alle genannten Therapieformen der HCL mit ihrer eingeschränkten myelopoietischen Funktion neu diskutiert werden müssen. Eine vorgezogene Rekonstitution der Hämopoiese könnte die Behandlungsmöglichkeiten der HCL stark beeinflussen.

Zunächst ist die praktische Seite der Anwendung des α-Ifns bei der HCL und die Ergebnisse in Bezug auf den erzielbaren Response zu besprechen.

Die geeignete Dosis hätte sich eskalierend erarbeitet werden sollen, wie es in der onkologischen Chemotherapie üblich ist. Dies ist bis heute nicht durchgeführt worden. Die Tagesdosis war früh niedrig gewählt worden. Das lag daran, daß 1983 das primär verwendete Leukozyten-Ifn (nIfn αle) nicht unbegrenzt zur Verfügung stand. Das schon niedrig gewählte Leukozyten-Ifn konnte noch durch pulsförmige Anwendung mit langen Pausen durch Clark et al. [8] erfolgreich verringert werden. Der Bericht von Clark gewann aber trotz interessanter Aspekte über intermittierende Induktionen mit Faktoren keine größere Bedeutung mehr, da schon zur gleichen Zeit im M. D. Anderson Hospital in Houston eine größere Patientengruppe mit dem eben gentechnologisch gewonnenen rekombinanten Ifn α-2a therapiert werden konnte [9]. Auch in anderen großen Zentren – u. a. von der länger mit der HCL beschäftigten Gruppe von Harvey Golomb – wurden jetzt Serien von Patienten mit humanen rekombinanten Interferonen (Ifn α-2b) begonnen [10]. Weltweit starteten weitere Therapiestudien. Neben gentechnologisch unbegrenzt herstellbaren wurde aus lymphoblastoiden Zellkulturen gewonnes Ifn n1 (Nawalma-Typ) mit einem α-Ifn-Anteil von ca. 35% in Großbritannien angewendet [11]. Seltener wurde das zweite Typ I-Ifn Ifn β aus Fibroblasten eingesetzt [12].

Früh war auch die 2- bis 3-malige Gabe in der Woche etabliert, sowie die subkutane Applikation. Sie war aus pharmakokinetischen Gründen für die α-Ifne übernommen worden. Allerdings waren nicht alle Studien sofort diesem Vorschlag gefolgt. Die subkutane Gabe setzte sich aber schnell durch, weil sie besonders gut den thrombopenischen HCL-Patienten entgegenkam, und sie war die Voraussetzung für die Eigeninjektion. Da aber trotz der geringen Dosen von 2–3 Millionen Einheiten pro Injektion (Bereich 0,2–3 Millionen) noch Nebenwirkungen auftraten, mußte die Suche nach der optimalen Dosis weitergehen. An die Thrombozytopenie adaptiert oder an Neopterin angepaßt arbeiteten sich zwei Gruppen an das Problem heran [13, 14]. Wir gingen in unserer Studiengruppe von einer niedrigen täglichen Dosis von 1,2 Millionen E/m^2 Ifn α-2c aus, die bei einem großen Teil unserer Patienten reduziert werden konnte, weil bei ihnen schon während der Induktionsphase von 84 Tagen an den Tagen 28 oder 56 eine deutliche Verbesserung der Blutwerte eingetreten war. In der Folge hatte mehr als die Hälfte unserer Patienten die Dosis während der damals noch so genannten Induktionsphase reduziert [15]. Die tägliche Applikation war gewählt worden, um eine nebenwirkungsarme Einzeldosis und einen kontinuierlichen Medikamentenspiegel zu erreichen, der weniger immunogen sein sollte. Zwei praktisch relevante Beobachtungen wurden während dieser multizentrischen Studie in mehr als 40 Kliniken mit über 90 Patienten gemacht. Zunächst verbesserte die tägliche Applikation die Abwehrleistung gefährdeter Patienten nicht ausreichend schnell, um sie vor tödlichen Infektionen zu schützen. Eher schien die kontinuierliche Beeinflussung des Abwehrsystems dessen spezifisch geforderte Infektionsabwehrleistung zu vermindern. Besonders splenektomierte Patienten erlitten tödliche Infektionen. Auch vermied die niedrige tägliche Dosis nicht sicher neuropsychiatrische Nebenwirkungen (3/91 Patienten).

Um die Hypothese von der Beeinträchtigung der Abwehr bei HCL-Patienten durch tägliches Ifn-α prüfen zu können, schlossen wir über die vergangenen 2 Jahre eine Studie an, die die als sicher und nicht infektionsgefährdet erschienenen Patienten ohne vorherige Splenektomie randomisiert der kontinuierlichen oder einer strikt pulsatilen Therapie unterwarfen. Als sich der Trend abzeichnete, daß auch für die primär behandelten Patienten unter pulsatiler Therapie die Sicherheit besser war, beendeten wir die Studie. Es hatten sich nämlich zwei Todesfälle während kontinuierlicher Therapie ereignet und einer in der Gruppe der pulsatil behandelten Patienten nach Einsetzen der zweimal wöchentlichen kontinuierlichen Erhaltungstherapie (noch nicht publiziert). Tatsächlich war die tägliche Applikation nicht notwendig. Nach vorläufiger Auswertung war die pulsatile Therapie in Bezug auf die Jansen-Stadien (d. h. die hämatologischen Parameter des Bluts) und den Karnofsky-Index (d. h. die Leistungsfähigkeit des Patienten) nicht wesentlich unterlegen. Die optimale Dosis und Pulsdauer sowie angepaßte Intervalle müssen noch erarbeitet werden. Über eine möglicherweise erhöhte Rate an induzierten Antikörpern ist noch nichts bekannt.

Ergebnisse

Die Tabelle 1 zeigt die Ansprechraten in allen größeren Studien. Sie übertreffen alle bekannten Daten zur Therapie niedrigmaligner Non-Hodgkin Lymphome. Zur feineren Analyse muß auf die Originalliteratur verwiesen werden.

Der Überblick über die weltweiten Studien läßt erkennen, daß inzwischen viele Patienten mit HCL eine Lebensqualität zurückerlangten, wie sie bisher nur vergleichbar ist mit der der insulinabhängigen, sehr gut eingestellten Diabetiker. Die Applikation ist dabei komfortabler und freier zu dosieren. Spätschäden sind noch nicht beschrieben. Stattdessen weicht die schleichende Gefahr der tödlichen Infektionen nach wenigen Monaten. Nur in einzelnen Fällen mit hohem Rsisiko und besonders unter täglicher Applikation scheint ihre Gefährlichkeit kurzfristig verstärkt [10].

Ergänzende Beobachtungen aus den Studien können Schlüssel zu neuen Anwendungsformen sein. Einige sollten deshalb angeführt werden.

1. Die Wiederherstellung der hämopoietischen Kapazität erfolgt unerklärterweise früher als das Schwinden der Haarzellen, das in vielen Fällen auch unvollständig bleibt oder erst nach 1–3 Jahren Therapie eintritt. Hier verhält sich Interferon wie ein Supplement, das mehr die negative Wirkung der HCL aufhebt, als die HCL verdrängt. Als Folge müssen wir akzeptieren, daß das primäre Therapieziel, nämlich die Wiederherstellung des Wohlbefindens, erreicht wird, ohne daß dabei der klassische Meßparameter der kompletten Remission eingetreten ist.

2. Die Zeiten bis zum Verschwinden der HC sind länger als bei konventioneller Therapie durch z. B. die einfache ablative Splenektomie, aber auch als bei der noch zu beschreibenden Therapie mit Deoxicoformycin.

3. Eine Resistenzentwicklung gegen Ifn im engeren Sinn wurde bisher nicht beobachtet.

Erhaltungstherapie

Die Langzeittherapie wird inzwischen für viele Patienten benötigt und ihre sichere Durchführbarkeit ist für den nicht kurativ behandelten Patienten von großer Bedeutung. Sie wird heute meistens mit zwei wöchentlichen Injektionen von 0,2 bis zu 2–3 Millionen α-Ifn s.c. durchgeführt. In dieser Form treten nur wenige unerwünschte Begleitreaktionen auf. Trotzdem wurden auch Auslaßversuche durchgeführt. Je nach vorher erreichter Remissionsqualität wurde erneute Therapiebedürftigkeit erst nach 6 bis über 18 Monaten beschrieben [16]. Fast alle Patienten sprachen bei Bedarf erneut an. Nicht bekannt ist, ob auch die 5–15% ganz von Haarzellen befreiten Patienten mit oder ohne Splenektomie eine solche Therapie benötigen. Die permanent selbsterhaltende komplette Remission würde einiges zur Biologie der HCL aussagen können.

Nebenwirkungen

Die hier erstmals mit einem gentechnologisch hergestellten Zytokin durchgeführte langfristige Therapie führt zur Entwicklung von Antikörpern gegen das Eiweiß. Sowohl Unregelmäßigkeiten der Tertiärstruktur und fehlende Glykosilierung wie in jedem Präparat ein anderer Austausch einzelner Aminosäuren können zur Antikörperbildung anregen. Wichtig werden wahrscheinlich nur die wirkungsneutralisierenden Antikörper. Die Neutralisation der antileukämischen Wirkung scheint aber nur wenig mit der Aufhebung der Kapazität zur Virusneutralisation parallel zu gehen [17]. Wirkungsneutralisierende Antikörper sind nicht häufig. Treten sie auf, können sie je nach Angriffspunkt überwunden werden. Antikörper gegen die Folgen der Punktmutationen und Strukturfehler können durch Umsetzen auf ein anderes rekombinantes Ifn $\alpha 2$ umgangen werden. Der fehlende Glykosilschutz muß durch Übergang auf natürliches Leukozyteninterferon (oder wahrscheinlich auch auf das α-Ifn, das aus lymphoblastoiden Namalvazellen gewonnen wird), überspielt werden. In ihm kommen mehrere verschiedene α-Interferone vor, die von der humanen Zelle glykosiliert hergestellt werden. Der denkbare Übergang auf das zweite Typ 1-Ifn, β-Ifn, das am selben Rezeptor wirkt, ist noch nicht beschrieben worden. Seine andere Pharmakokinetik und möglicherweise die Wirkung des Begleitproteins aus den Fibroblasten B-Zell-Wachstumsfaktor (BCGF oder β-Ifn 2), der die Regression der HCL verhindern könnte, gestalten den Einsatz zur Zeit noch unübersichtlich [12]. Neben den schwerwiegenden, die Effizienz bedrohenden Antikörpern sind in der Langzeittherapie auch geringere unerwünschte Begleitreaktionen zu beachten. Minimale depressive Verstimmungen und Behinderungen des Tagesablaufs summieren sich. Meistens führt die Eigenapplikation zu geschickten Lösungen durch die Patienten. Sie nutzen dann die Eigenheiten ihres Tagesablaufs, um ihre Begleitreaktion in die Ruhephase zu verlagern. Die Injektion am frühen Nachmittag hilft vielen, den folgenden Morgen frisch zu beginnen. Die Injektion am späten Nachmittag verlegt die 4–5 h später einsetzende Frierreaktion vieler Patienten auf die Zeit des Schlafengehens. Der geschickte Umgang mit Dosissteigerung nach niedrigdosiertem Beginn und die geringe Rate an Nebenwirkungen erlaubten die Primärtherapie mit α-Ifn auch im höheren Alter. Eine Splenektomie ist nicht Voraussetzung. Es lohnt sich, auch in der Dauertherapie die Dosen bei älteren Patienten niedrig (z. B. unter 500 000 IE U/Tag) zu wählen. Auch Therapiepausen scheinen für eine palliative Therapie alter Patienten sinnvoll.

Für jüngere Patienten wird jetzt aber Kuration angestrebt. Erst dadurch werden dauerhaft Infektionen und Begleitreaktionen wie Antikörperbildung vermieden. Die Fähigkeit des α-Ifns, anhaltende Remissionen auch noch nach mehreren Jahren zu erzielen, ist noch unbestimmt, aber möglich. Die Kriterien für den Response wurden zunächst nur aus Kurzzeitbeobachtungen abgeleitet und an den physiologischen Ablauf der Zell-«mauserung» adaptiert. Für die Verbesserung bleiben jetzt noch folgende offene Fragen: Muß die Zellmasse vor der Therapie durch Splenektomie reduziert werden [18]? Ich glaube nicht. Nach den Daten über die sIL2R scheint der Unterschied in der Zellmasse nicht groß [19].

Die Aufarbeitung solcher Fragen mag heute durch zwei neue Parameter des Ansprechens der HCL erleichtert werden. Die Haarzellen tragen eine große Zahl von Interleukin 2-Rezeptoren (Il 2R). Jetzt kann ein löslicher Abkömmling im Serum gemessen werden (sIL2-R) [20]. Damit steht eine neue Meßmethode für den Restbestand an Haarzellen zur Verfügung. Zu diesem Parameter gesellt sich die Beobachtung, daß die serumständigen Derivate des CD8-Antigens der T-Suppressor-Zellen (SCD8) sich unter der Therapie mit Interferon zur Normalität hin bewegen [19]. Die biologische Bedeutung dieses Phänomens ist nicht erhellt. Aber die oben genannte Infektionsanfälligkeit während kontinuierlicher Therapie könnte damit in Verbindung gebracht werden. Der Befund ist durch veränderte Immunglobulinsynthese und die reduzierte Granulozytenfunktion zu ergänzen [21]. Sie können hier nicht weiter diskutiert werden. Diese meist zwar untergeordneten, aber mannigfachen negativen Einflüsse des Ifns auf die Abwehrfunktion läßt den zeitlich gekoppelten Einsatz von Wachstumsstimulatoren bedenken.

Aussichten

Eine drastische Zellreduktion der HCL ist durch Deoxicoformycin (DCF), einen Hemmer der Adenosindesaminase, möglich geworden. Diese Substanz führt bei der HCL sehr oft allein zu langanhaltenden sogenannten kompletten Remissionen. Sollte die Ifn-Therapie die Zellmauserung bis zur Heilung fortsetzen können, so sollte es die Zytoreduktion einleiten, die durch α-Ifn stabilisiert würde. Erste Auswertungen von wenigen Patienten trüben aber schon die Aussichten auf die Addierbarkeit der Substanzen [23]. So erscheinen wie so oft in der Therapie hinter den Erfolgen in der Remissionsinduktion neue Fragen zur Langzeitbehandlung. Wir sind aufgerufen, auf eine Lösung hinzuwirken. Obwohl das Schicksal der Patienten in weniger als 5 Jahren erfolgreich durch α-Ifn gewendet werden konnte, müssen wir die Herausforderung annehmen und uns auf eine neue Ära nach der Etablierung der Ifn-Therapie einstellen.

Danksagung

Viele Beobachtungen verdanke ich Kollegen, die an zwei kooperativen multizentrischen Studien in der BRD teilgenommen haben. Die Studien waren ermöglicht von den Firmen Dr. Karl Thomae und Hoffmann-La Roche, die Berofor[A] und Roferon[A] stellten.

Literatur

1 Anderson, K.C.; Bolyd, A.W.; Fisher, D. C.; Leslie, D.; Schlossmann, S.F.; Adler, L.M.: Hairy cell leukemia: A tumor of preplasma cells. Blood *65:* 620–629 (1985).

2 Seshadri, R.S.; Brown, E.J.; Zipurski, A.: Leukemic reticuloendotheliosis: A failure of monocyte production. New Engl. J. Med. *295:* 181 (1976).

3 Flandrin, G.; Sigaux, F.; Castaigne, S.; Calvo, F.; Sebahoun, G.; Glot, P.: Leucemie a tricholeucocytes: etude d'evolution de 211 cas. Nouv. Press Med. *13:* 2795–2799 (1984).

4 Quesada, J.R.; Hersh, E.M.; Gutterman, J.U.: Biologic therapy of hairy cell leukemia. Semin. Oncol. *11:* 507 (1984).

5 Sigaux, F.; Castaigne, S.; Lehn, P.; Dupuy, W.; Billard, C.; Gluckman, J.-C.; Boiron, M.; Falcoff, E.; Flandrin, G.; Degos, L.: Alpha-interferon in hairy cell leukemia: Direct effects on hairy cells or indirect cytotoxicity? Int. J. Cancer *1:* 2–8 (1987).

6 Steis, R. G.; Smith, J. W.; Urba, W. J.; Clark, J. W.; Loretta, M.I.; Evans, L.M.; Schoenberger, C.; Longo, D.L.: Resistance to recombinant interferon alfa-2a in hairy cell leukemia associated with neutralizing anti-interferon antibodies. New Engl. J. Med. *318:* 1409–1413 (1988).

7 Donahue, R.E.; Wang, E.A. et al.: Stimulation of hematopoiesis in primates by continuous infusion of human GM-CSF. Natur *321:* 872–875 (1986).

8 Clark, R.; Dimitrov, N.; Axelson, J.; Penner, J.; Oviatt, D.: Low dose intermittent IFn in the treatment of hairy cell leukemia. Proc. Am. Soc. clin. Oncol. *4:* 161–626 (1985).

9 Quesada, J.R.; Gutterman, J.U.; Hersh, E.M.: Treatment of hairy cell leukemia with alpha interferons. Cancer *57:* 1678–1680 (1986).

10 Golomb, H.M.: The treatment of hairy cell leukemia. Blood *69:* 979–983 (1987).

11 Worman, C.P.; Nethersell, A.B.; Bottomley, J.M.; Apostolow, K.; Barker, W.; Cawley, J.C.: Natural interferon alpha therapy in hairy cell leukemia (namalva-type IFn – Wellferon). Klin. Wschr. *65:* 685–687 (1987).

12 Wussow, P. von; Düllmann, J.; Grethlein, T.; Hirschmann, W.D.; Hügl, E.; Koch, O.; Martin, W.R.; Pees, H.W.; Urbanitz, W.; Freund, M.; IFN-β-Therapie bei der Haarzell-Leukämie. Klin. Wschr. *65:* 688–690 (1987).

13 Porzsolt, F.; Thomä, J.; Unsöld, M.; Wolf, W.; Obert, H.J.; Kubanek, B.; Heimpel, H.: Platelet adjusted IFn-dosage in the treatment of advanced hairy cell leukemia. Blut *51:* 73–82 (1985).

14 Gastl, G.; Lang, A.; Huber, C.H.; Seewann, H.: Interferon-alpha for idiopathic myelofibrosis. Lancet *ii:* 8588 765–766 (1988).

15 Pralle, H.; Zwingers, Th. et al.: A prospective multicenter trial with human recombinant alpha 2c-Interferon in hairy cell leukemia before and after splenectomy. Leukemia *1:* 337–340 (1987).

16 Ratain, M.; Golomb, H.; Bardawol, R.G.; Vardiman, J.; Westbrook, C.A.; Kaminer, L.S.; Lembersky, B.C.; Bitter, M.A.; Daly, K.: Durability of responses to Interferon-α2b in advanced hairy cell leukemia. Blood *69:* 872–877 (1987).

17 Steis, R.G.; Foon, K.A.; Longo, D.: Current and future uses of recombinant interferon alpha in the treatment of low-grade Non-Hodgkins's lymphoma. Cancer *59:* 658–663 (1987).

18 Golomb, H.M.; Fefer, A.; Golde, D.W.; Ozer, H.; Portlock, C.; Silber, R.; Rappeport, J.; Ratain, M.J.; Thompson, J.; Bonnem, E.M.; Spiegel, R.J.; Tensen, L.; Burke, J.S.; Vardiman, J.W.: Sequential evaluation of alpha-2b-Interferon treatment in 128 patients with hairy cell leukemia. Semin. Oncol. *14:* 13–17 (1987).

19 Ho, A.D.; Großmann, M.; Knauf, W.; Martin, H.; Zwingers, Th.; Trümper, L.; Sonnen, R.; Pralle, H.; Hunstein, W.: Plasma levels of SCD_8 and sIC 2-R in patients with hairy cell leukemia, relationship with splenectomy and with clinical response to therapy (eingereicht).

20 Chilosi, B.M.; Semenzato, G.C. et al.: Soluble interleukin-2 receptors in the sera of patients with hairy cell leukemia: Relationship with the effect of recombinant alpha-Interferon therapy on clinical parameters and natural killer in vitro activity. Blood *70:* 1530–1535 (1987).

21 Harfast, B.; Huddlestone, J.R.; Casaili, P.; Merigan, T.C.; Oldstone, M.B.A.: Interferon acts directly on human B-lymphocytes to modulate immunoglobulin synthesis. J. Immunol. *127:* 2146–2150 (1981).

22 Ernstoff, M.S.; Gallichio, V.; Kirkwood, J.M.: Analysis of granulocyte-macrophage progenitor cells in patients treated with recombinant interferon alpha 2. Am. J. Med. *79:* 167–170 (1985).

23 Nerenstone, S.; Martin, A.; Urba, W.; Lawrence, J.; Clark, J.; Smith, J.; Crum, E.; Miller, R.; Schoenberger, C.; Hawkins, M.; Longo, D.; Steis, R.: Treatment of hairy cell leukemia (HCL) with alternating cycles of 2'deoxycoformycin (DCF) and recombinant alpha-2a interferon (IFN). Proc. ASCO Clin. Oncol. *7:* 729 (1988).

24 Schwarzmeier, J.D.; Wagner, L.; Prischl, F.; Schwabe, M.; Lion, T.; Micksche, M.; Köller, U.; Bernhart, M.; Fritz, O.; Sewann, H.L.; Michlmayr, G.: Rekombinante (IFN-α_{2b})-Therapie der Haarzell-Leukämie. Klin. Wschr. *65:* 699–705 (1987).

25 Glaspy, J.A.; Jacobs, A.D.; Golde, D.W.: The Ucla experience with type I interferons in hairy cell leukemia. Leukemia *1:* 323–326 (1987).

26 Castaigne, S.; Sigaux, F.; Cantell, K.; Falcoff, E.; Boiron, M.; Flandrin, G.; Degos, L.: Interferon alpha in the treatment of hairy cell leukemia. Cancer *57:* 1681–1684 (1986).

Prof. Dr. H. Pralle, Abteilung Hämatologie/Onkologie, Medizinische Kliniken der Justus-Liebig-Universität Gießen, Klinikstraße 36, D-6300 Gießen (BRD)

Beitr Onkol, vol. 36, pp. 106–115 (Karger, Basel 1989)

Die Rolle von Tumornekrosefaktor bei der Wachstumsregulation von B-Zell-Malignomen

F. Porzsolt, Ch. Buck, W. Digel, H. Heimpel

Abteilung Innere Medizin III, Universität Ulm

Einleitung

Tumornekrosefaktor-α (TNF-α), der von Makrophagen und Lymphozyten produziert wird, hat als potentielle antitumorale Substanz Bedeutung gewonnen, da dieser Faktor für verschiedene Tumoren zytotoxisch ist und in vitro zu hämorraghischen Tumornekrosen führt [1, 2]. Die Aufklärung der Struktur ergab eine Homologie von 30% mit dem Zytokin TNF-β, welches von aktivierten T-Zellen produziert wird [3]. Beide Zytokine binden am gleichen spezifischen Rezeptor und vermitteln ähnliche biologische Aktivitäten. So wurde gezeigt, daß TNF-α die Phagozytose polymorphkerniger Zellen und deren Adhärenz an Endothelzellen steigert [4, 5]; es induziert die Produktion von Zytokinen [6–8], verstärkt die Expression von HLA-Antigenen [9] und hat antivirale Eigenschaften [10]. Neben der antitumoralen Wirkung kann TNF-α auch das Wachstum von Fibroblasten [11], T-Zellen [12] und Thymozyten [13] steigern. In neueren Arbeiten wurde gezeigt, daß die DNA-Synthese aktivierter B-Lymphozyten von gesunden Spendern durch TNF-α stimuliert werden kann [14]. Auch TNF-β steigert die Proliferation aktivierter B-Zellen [15]. Am Beispiel von Osteosarkomzellen wurde beschrieben, daß TNF auch bei malignen Zellen zu einer Stimulation des Wachstums führen kann [16].

Im vorliegenden Beitrag wird untersucht, ob TNF das Wachstum maligner B-Zellen von Patienten mit Haarzell-Leukämie (HCL) und chronisch lymphatischer Leukämie (CLL) beeinflussen kann.

Patienten und Methoden

Patienten

In die Studie wurden gesunde Kontrollpersonen, Patienten mit Haarzell-Leukämie vor und nach Therapie sowie unbehandelte Patienten mit CLL eingeschlossen. Die Diagnosen stützten sich auf klinische Befunde, morphologische Untersuchung des peripheren Blutes und von Knochenmarksbiopsien, Immunphänotypisierung und auf histologische Befunde der Milz bei splenektomierten Haarzell-Leukämie-Patienten. Nach vorliegender Zustimmung wurde heparinisiertes peripheres Blut abgenommen.

Trennung der Zellen

Mononukleäre Zellen (MNC) wurden nach Trennung über einem Ficoll-Hypaque-Gradienten (Pharmacie, Freiburg) gewonnen. Zur Gewinnung von Haarzellen und CLL-Zellen wurden adhärente Monozyten durch Inkubation der MNC in Plastik-Flaschen (Nunc, Wiesbaden) über 90 min bei 38 °C in RPMI 1640 Medium (Gibco, Karlsruhe) mit 10% FCS entfernt. Aus den verbleibenden Zellen wurden die T-Zellen durch Rosettierung mit Neuraminidase behandelten Schaferythrozyten entfernt. Die nicht-rosettierenden Zellen wurden durch einen zweiten Ficoll-Hypaque-Gradienten abgetrennt. Der Anteil der B-Zellen, residualen Monozyten und T-Zellen wurde durch indirekte Immunfluoreszenz bestimmt.

Immunfluoreszenz

Die Zellen wurden mit spezifischen monoklonalen Antikörpern mit der indirekten Immunfluoreszenz-Methode in Suspension markiert. Nach Inkubation über 30 min mit dem spezifischen Antikörper wurden die Zellen mit Fluoreszenz-isothiozyanat-konjugiertem Ziege anti Maus IgG oder IgM gefärbt und mit einem Immunfluoreszenz-Mikroskop beurteilt.

Reagentien

Hochgereinigter rTNF-α und rTNF-β wurden von BASF/Knoll, Mannheim, zur Verfügung gestellt. Die spezifische Aktivität von rTNF-α betrug 6.63×10^6 U/mg Protein und von rTNF-β $6 \times 10^<$ U/mg. Polyklonale Antikörper gegen rTNF-α und rTNF-β wurden uns vom Ernst-Boehringer-Institut für Arzneimittelforschung, Wien, überlassen.

DNS-Sythese

Die DNS-Syntheserate wurde durch die Thymidin (^{3}H-TdR) Aufnahme bestimmt. Gereinigte Populationen von Haarzellen und CLL-Zellen wurden in 96-Loch-Mikrotiter-Platten mit flachem Boden (Nunc, Wiesbaden) in Triplikaten (6×10^5 Zellen) kultiviert. Weniger als 5%

der Zellen wurden durch Trypan Blau angefärbt. Rekombinanter TNF-α oder TNF-β wurden in Konzentrationen zwischen 1 und 100 ng/ml zugegeben. Die Zellen wurden bis zu 144 h bei 37 °C in 5% CO_2 und 98% Luftfeuchtigkeit in RPMI 1640 mit 10% hitzeinaktiviertem FCS inkubiert. Sieben h vor Ende der Kultur wurde 1 uCi ^{3}H-Thymidin (6,7 Ci/mMol, Amersham, Braunschweig) zugegeben. Der ^{3}H-Einbau wurde im Liquid Scintillation Counter gemessen. Der Stimulations-Index ist als Quotient der stimulierten/nicht-stimulierten Proben angegeben.

TNF-Induktion in vitro

MNC von gesunden Kontrollpersonen und Patienten mit Haarzell-Leukämie sowie gereinigte Haarzellen wurden mit PHA (Wellcome, Burgwedel) und 4β-phorbol 12β-myristat 13-acetat (TPA, Sigma Chemicals, Freiburg) 8 und 48 h induziert. Die zytotoxische Aktivität in den zellfreien Überständen wurde im L-929-Assay bestimmt.

TNF-Bioassay

Zum Nachweis zytotoxischer Aktivität in zellfreien Kulturüberständen wurde der L-929 Fibroblasten-Lyse-Assay verwendet. Dazu wurden L-929 Zellen (5×10^4/Loch) in Miktrotiter-Platten mit flachem Boden zusammen mit serienmäßig verdünnten Testproben 18 h bei 39,5 °C in Gegenwart von Actinomycin D (2 μg/ml) inkubiert. Die Platten wurden gewaschen und mit Kristallviolett (0,5%) gefärbt. Die zytotoxische Aktivität wurde anhand mitgeführter Standards für TNF-α und TNF-β bestimmt.

Ergebnisse

Spontane DNS-Synthese von Haarzellen und CLL-Zellen

Der spontane ^{3}H-TdR-Einbau betrug bei Haarzellen von 8 Patienten nach 48-h-Kultur im median 481 cpm (Bereich 458–1469) und stieg nach 120 h um den Faktor 1,3 bis 3,0.

Der spontane Einbau von CLL-Zellen betrug nach 48-h-Kultur im median 532 cpm (Bereich 351–1822). Nach 96 h wurde in 3/10 Fällen ein mehr als zweifacher Anstieg der spontanen DNA-Synthese beobachtet. Bei 7/10 Patienten war kein spontaner Anstieg der DNA-Synthese zu messen (Abb. 1).

Stimulation mit rekombinantem TNF-α

Nach Stimulation von Haarzellen wurde der maximale ^{3}H-TdR-Einbau mit 10 bis 25 ng/ml rTNF-α erreicht. Im untersuchten Zeitintervall (48–120 h) war bei einem Patienten der maximale Einbau bereits nach 48 h

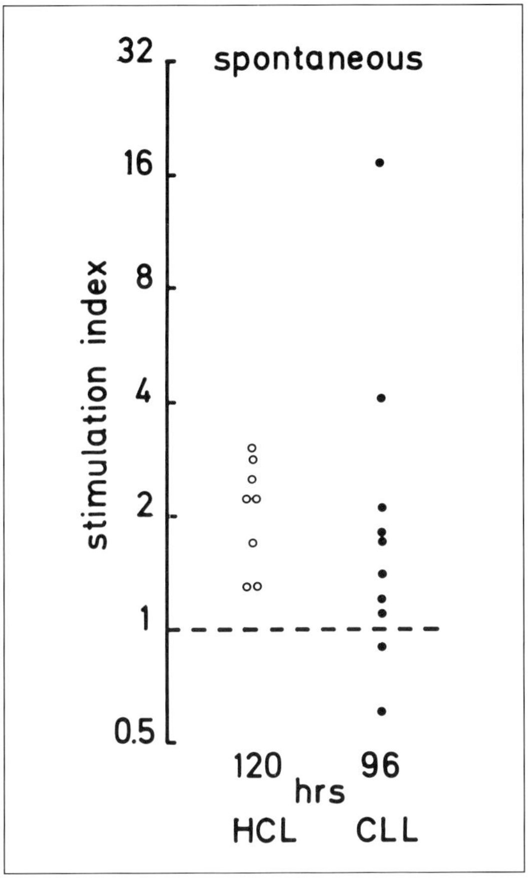

Abb. 1. Spontaner ³H-TdR-Einbau in gereinigten Haarzellen und B-Lymphozyten von Patienten mit CLL. Der Stimulationsindex beschreibt den Quotienten des ³H-TdR Einbaus nach 120 bzw. 96 h gegenüber 48-h-Kultur.

erreicht. Nach 120 h war der durch TNF-α induzierte ^{3}H-TdR-Einbau bei 5/8 Patienten gegenüber den unbehandelten Kontrollen auf mindestens das zweifache gesteigert (Abb. 2).

Die Stimulation mit rTNF-β (1–50 ng/ml) über 48–120 h zeigte keine signifikante Steigerung des ^{3}H-TdR-Einbaus gegenüber unstimulierten Kontrollen.

Bei CLL-Patienten war der maximale ^{3}H-TdR-Einbau ebenfalls mit 10–25 ng/ml TNF-α zu erzielen. Die DNA-Synthese erreichte bei CLL in der Regel nach 72 h ein Maximum, welches in den untersuchten Fällen auch nach Kultur über 144 h nicht weiter anstieg. Nach 48 h Kultur war die DNA-Synthese durch TNF in 3/10 Fällen gegenüber unbehandelten Kon-

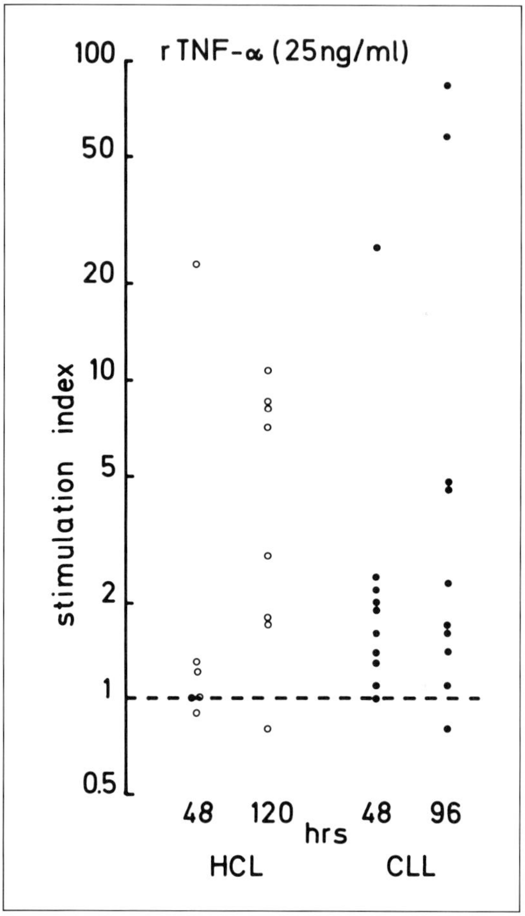

Abb. 2. ^{3}H-TdR-Einbau in gereinigten Haarzellen und B-Lymphozyten von Patienten mit CLL nach In-vitro-Stimulation mit rTNF-*α*. Der Stimulationsindex beschreibt den Quotienten des ^{3}H-TdR Einbaus mit/ohne rTNF-*α*.

trollen mehr als verdoppelt. Nach 96 h konnte bei 5/10 Patienten ein mehr als zweifacher Anstieg der DNA-Synthese nachgewiesen werden.

Zellwachstum nach Stimulation mit TNF

Bei drei untersuchten Patienten mit HCL konnten die Zellen über mehr als 50 Tage kultiviert werden. Die Viabilität betrug 70%. Allerdings kam es zu keinem signifikanten Anstieg der Zellzahl. In unbehandelten Kontrollen sank die Viabilität innerhalb von 20 Tagen auf 10% ab.

Bei CLL-Patienten ohne spontanes Wachstum wurde nach Kultur mit TNF-α über 120 h kein signifikanter Anstieg der Zellzahl beobachtet. In der entsprechenden Kultur unbehandelter Kontrollen sank die Zellzahl im gleichen Zeitraum auf 50% der Ausgangskonzentration ab. Somit war in TNF-stimulierten Kulturen zwar keine Zunahme der Zellen nachzuweisen; durch TNF konnte aber das Absterben der Kultur verhindert werden.

TNF-Produktion

Im Kulturüberstand mononukleärer Zellen von gesunden Kontrollpersonen konnte ohne Induktion in keinem von 10 Fällen zytotoxische Aktivität im L929-Assay nachgewiesen werden. Dagegen war in 2/9 HCL-Kulturen eine spontane Freisetzung geringer Mengen zytotoxischer Aktivität nachweisbar (Abb. 3). Nach Induktion mit PHA oder PHA+TPA über 8

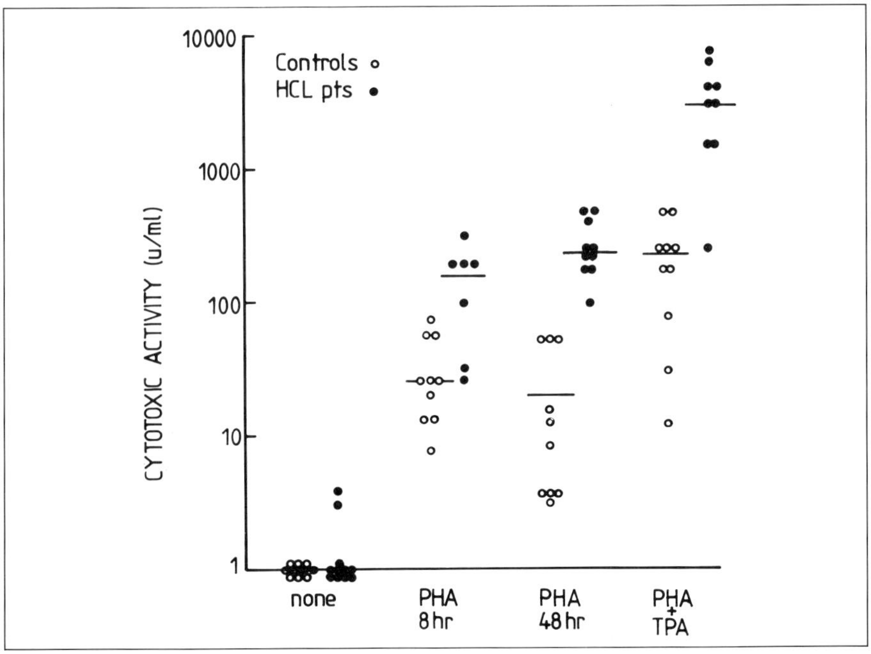

Abb. 3. In-vitro-Induktion zytotoxischer Aktivität ohne und mit PHA und TPA in mononukleären Zellen von gesunden Kontrollpersonen und Patienten mit Haarzell-Leukämie. Die zytotoxische Aktivität der Kulturüberstände wurde im L-929-Assay getestet und ist als Units/ml angegegen.

und 48 h produzierten mononukleäre Zellen von Patienten mit HCL etwa 10fach höhere Konzentrationen zytotoxischer Aktivität im Kulturüberstand als mononukleäre Zellen gesunder Spender (Abb. 3).

Ein Vergleich der PHA-induzierten zytotoxischen Aktivität vor Therapie bzw. nach Splenektomie oder Interferon-Therapie bestätigte im Vergleich zu gesunden Kontrollen die erhöhte Produktion zytotoxischer Aktivität durch Zellen unbehandelter Patienten. Nach Verminderung des Anteils der Haarzellen im peripheren Blut durch Splenektomie oder Therapie mit Interferon-α konnten nur geringe zytotoxische Aktivitäten wie in Zellen gesunder Kontrollen induziert werden (Tab. 1).

Diskussion

Die Stimulation maligner B-Zellen konnte bereits früher in vitro durch Interleukin-2 oder BCGF gezeigt werden [17, 18]. Unsere eigenen Ergebnisse sowie die Befunde anderer [19] demonstrieren, daß auch TNF das Wachstum maligner B-Zellen stimulieren kann. Der wachstumsstimulierende Effekt von TNF ist nicht spezifisch für maligne B-Zellen, da in früheren Arbeiten gezeigt wurde, daß das Wachstum von B-Zellen gesunder Spender, allerdings nach vorausgegangener In-vitro-Aktivierung, durch TNF-α stimuliert werden kann [14]. Es ist unwahrscheinlich, daß die induzierte DNA-Synthese durch eine Kontamination des rekombinanten Zytokins mit Endotoxin erfolgte, da der stimulierende Effekt von rTNF vollständig durch einen Antikörper gegen TNF inhibiert werden konnte. Allerdings ist nicht geklärt,

Tabelle 1. In-vitro-Induktion zytotoxischer Aktivität mit PHA in mononukleären Zellen von gesunden Kontrollpersonen und Patienten mit Haarzell-Leukämie vor und nach Therapie. Die zytotoxische Aktivität der Kulturüberstände wurde im L-929-Assay getestet. Mittelwerte ± Standardabweichung sind dargestellt

	n	zytotoxische Aktivität (U/ml) $x \pm s$
Gesunde Kontrollen	10	23 ± 20
HCL vor Therapie	11	212 ± 153
HCL nach IFN-α	9	48 ± 32
HCL nach Splenektomie	7	29 ± 32

ob der wachstumsstimulierende Effekt durch TNF-α oder über die Induktion weiterer Zytokine vermittelt wird, da das Wachstum maligner B-Zellen auch durch IL-2 [17] und BCGF [18] gesteigert werden konnte. Außerdem gibt es Hinweise, daß die Sensitivität gegenüber TNF durch verschiedene Zytokine moduliert werden kann [20].

Die Bedeutung von TNF-β bei der Wachstumsregulation maligner B-Zellen ist bisher nicht geklärt. Einerseits konnte durch rekombinantes TNF-β in keinem Fall das Wachstum maligner B-Zellen induziert werden; andererseits war in früheren Experimenten bei Haarzell-Leukämie der wachstumsstimulierende Effekt von PHA-konditioniertem Medium durch Zugaben eines Antikörpers gegen TNF-β, nicht jedoch durch Zugabe eines Antikörpers gegen TNF-α, zu inhibieren [21].

Es gibt mehrere Hinweise, daß Zytokine und namentlich TNF bei Patienten mit B-Zell-Malignomen in vivo produziert werden. In eigenen Untersuchungen wurde eine spontane Produktion zytotoxischer Faktoren beobachtet, wenn mononukleäre Zellen von Patienten mit Haarzell-Leukämie, nicht jedoch von gesunden Spendern, kultiviert wurden. Einer britischen Arbeitsgruppe war es gelungen, die spezifische m-RNA aus gereinigten Haarzellen eines Patienten nachzuweisen [19]. Dieses Signal konnte durch vorherige Behandlung mit rekombinantem TNF-α verstärkt werden. Diese positive Rückkopplung wurde auch an HL60-Zellen nachgewiesen [22]. Außerdem konnten wir mit einem spezifischen ELISA für TNF-α Spuren dieses Zytokins in einigen Seren von Patienten mit Haarzell-Leukämie nachweisen.

Wir konnten an HCL-Patienten zeigen, daß mit einer Verminderung der Haarzellen im peripheren Blut, die durch Splenektomie oder Interferon-α-Therapie erreicht wurde, auch die in MNC induzierte zytotoxische Aktivität vermindert war. Dieser Befund zeigt, daß neben T-Zellen auch HCL-Zellen als Produzenten der zytotoxischen Aktivität zu diskutieren sind. Diese Annahme wird durch den Nachweis der m-RNA für TNF-α in HCL-Zellen gestützt [19].

Anmerkungen

Unser Dank gilt BASF/Knoll sowie dem Ernst-Boehringer-Institut für Arzneimittelforschung für die Überlassung der Reagentien. Frau S. Scholz sind wir für die sorgfältige technische Unterstützung zu Dank verpflichtet. Frau I. Brand danken wir für die Hilfe bei der Fertigstellung des Manuskripts.

Literatur

1 Old, L.J.: Tumor necrosis factor (TNF). Science *230:* 630–632 (1985).

2 Sugarman, B.J.; Aggarwal, B.B.; Hass, P.E.; Figari, I.S.; Palladino, M.A., Jr.; Shepard, H.M.: Recombinant human tumor necrosis factor-alpha: effects on proliferation of normal and transformed cells in vitro. Science *230:* 943–945 (1985).

3 Cuturi, M.C.; Murphy, M.; Costa-Giomi, M.P.; Weinmann, R.; Perussia, B.; Trinchieri, G.: Independent regulation of tumor necrosis factor and lymphotoxin production by human peripheral blood lymphocytes. J. Exp. Med. *165:* 1581–1594 (1987).

4 Shalaby, M.R.; Aggarwal, B.B.; Rinderknecht, E.; Sverdersky, L.P.; Finkle, B.S.; Palladino, M.A. Jr.: Activation of human polymorphonucelar neutrophil functions by interferon-gamma and tumor necrosis factor. J. Immunol. *135:* 2069–2073 (1985).

5 Gamble, J.R.; Harlan, J.M.; Klebanoff, S.J.; Vadas, M.A.: Stimulation of the adherence of neutrophils to umbilical vein endothelium by human recombinant tumor necrosis factor. Proc. Natl. Acad. Sci. USA *82:* 8667–8671 (1985).

6 Oster, W.; Lindemann, A.; Horn, S.; Mertelsmann, R.; Herrmann, F.: Tumor necrosis factor (TNF)-alpha but not TNF-beta induces secretion of colony stimulating factor for macrophages (CSF-1) by human monocytes. Blood *70:* 1700–1703 (1987).

7 Locksley, R.M.; Heinzel, F.P.; Shepard, H.M.; Agosti, J.; Eessaulu, T.E.; Aggarwal, B.B.; Harlan, J.M.: Tumor necrosis factors α und β differ in their capacities to generate Interleukin 1 release from human endothelial cells. J. Immunol. *139:* 1891–1895 (1987).

8 Koeffler, H.P.; Gasson, J.; Ranyard, J.; Souza, L.; Shepard, M.; Munker, R.: Recombinant human TNF-α stimulates production of granulocyte colony-stimulating factor. Blood *70:* 55–59 (1987).

9 Pfizenmaier, K.; Scheurich, P.; Schlüter, C.; Krönke, M.: Tumor necrosis factor enhances HLA-A, B. C and HLA-DR gene expression in human tumor cells. J. Immunol. *138:* 975–980 (1987).

10 Mestan, J.; Digel, W.; Mittnach, S.; Hillen, H.; Blohm, D.; Möller, A.; Jacobsen, H.; Kirchner, H.: Antiviral effects of recombinant tumour necrosis factor in vitro. Natur *323:* 816–822 (1986).

11 Vilcek, J.; Palombella, V.J.; Henriksen-De Stafano, D.; Swenson, C.,; Feinman, R.; Hirai, M.; Tsujimoto, M.: Fibroblast growth enhancing activity of tumor necrosis factor and its relationship to other polypeptide growth factors. J. Exp. Med. *163:* 632–643 (1986).

12 Zucali, J.R.; Elfenbein, G.J.; Barth, K.C.; Dinarello, C.A.: Effects of human Il-1 and human TNF on human T lymphocyte colony formation. J. Clin. Invest. *80:* 772–777 (1987).

13 Ranges, G.E.; Zlotnik, A.; Espevik, T.; Dinarello, C.A.; Cerami, A.; Palladino, M.A.: Tumor necrosis factor alpha/cachectin is a growth factor for thymocytes. J. Exp. Med. *176:* 1472–1478 (1988).

14 Kehrl, J.H.; Miller, A.; Fauci, A.S.: Effect of TNF alpha on mitogen activated human B cells. J. Exp. Med. *166:* 786–791 (1987).

15 Kehrl, J.H.; Alvarez-Mon, M.; Delsing, G.A.; Fauci, A.S.: Lymphotoxin is an important T cellderived growth factor for human B cells. Science *238:* 1144–1146 (1987).

16 Kirstein, M.; Baglioni, C.: Mitogenic activity of tumor necrosis factor for human osteosarcoma cells; in Immunobiology, p. 64, Vol. 175, No. 1/2 (Fischer, Stuttgart 1987).

17 Karray, S.; Merle-Beral, H.; Vazques, A.; Gerard, J.P.; Debre, P.; Galanaud, P.: Functional heterogeneity of B-CLL lymphocytes: dissociated responsiveness to growth factors and distinct requirements for a first activation signal. Blood *70:* 1105–1110 (1987).

18 Paganelli, K.S.; Evans, S.S.; Han, T.; Ozer, H.: B cell growth factor-induced proliferation of hairy cell lymphocytes and inhibition by type I interferon in vitro. Blood *67:* 937–942 (1986).

19 Cordingley, F.T.; Hoffbrand, a.V.; Heslop, H.E.; Turner, M.; Bianchi, A.; Reittie, J.E.; Vyakarnam, A.; Meager, A.; Brenner, M.K.: Tumor necrosis factor as an autocrine tumour growth factor for chronic B-cell malignancies. Lancet *i:* 969–971 (1988).

20 Pfizenmaier, K.; Krönke, M.; Scheurich, P.; Nagel, G.A.: Tumor necrosis factor (TNF) alpha: control of TNF-sensitivity and molecular mechanisms of TNF-mediated growth inhibition. Blut *53:* 1–10 (1987).

21 Porzsolt, F.; Digel, W.; Buck, C.; Raghavachar, A.; Stefanic, M.; Schöniger, W.: Possible mechanism of Interferon action in hairy cell leukemia; in Beger, New approaches in cancer therapy (Springer, Berlin, im Druck).

22 Hensel, G.; Männel, D.N.; Pfizenmaier, K.; Krönke, M.: Autocrine stimulation of TNF-alpha mRNA expression in HL-60 cells. Lymphokine Res. (im Druck).

PD Dr. F. Porzsolt, Abt. Innere Medizin III, Universität Ulm,
Oberer Eselsberg, Robert-Koch-Str. 8, D-7900 Ulm (BRD)